Zoonosis of Public Health Interest

Edited by Gilberto Bastidas

Published in London, United Kingdom

Zoonosis of Public Health Interest
http://dx.doi.org/10.5772/intechopen.100934
Edited by Gilberto Bastidas

Contributors
Moses Adriko, Sabina Seric-Haracic, Jasmin Omeragic, Naida Kapo, Jitendrakumar Bhogilal Nayak, Jeetendrakumar Harnathbhai Chaudhary, Urvish Pravinbhai Mistry, Prakrutik Prafulchandra Bhavsar, Manojbhai N. Brahmbhatt, Pranav Ashok Anjaria, Timothy J. Tse, Farley Chicilo, Jeffrey Popiel, Martin J.T. Reaney, Gilberto Bastidas, Andrew W. Taylor-Robinson, Olaitan O. Omitola, Roy D. Meléndez, Sinforiano J. Posadas, Fernando José Ojeda, Maria Gabriela Barreto Costa De Matos

First published in London, United Kingdom, 2022 by IntechOpen
IntechOpen is the global imprint of INTECHOPEN LIMITED, registered in England and Wales, registration number: 11086078, 5 Princes Gate Court, London, SW7 2QJ, United Kingdom

British Library Cataloguing-in-Publication Data
A catalogue record for this book is available from the British Library

Additional hard and PDF copies can be obtained from orders@intechopen.com

Zoonosis of Public Health Interest
Edited by Gilberto Bastidas
p. cm.
Print ISBN 978-1-80356-113-4
Online ISBN 978-1-80356-114-1
eBook (PDF) ISBN 978-1-80356-115-8

Meet the editor

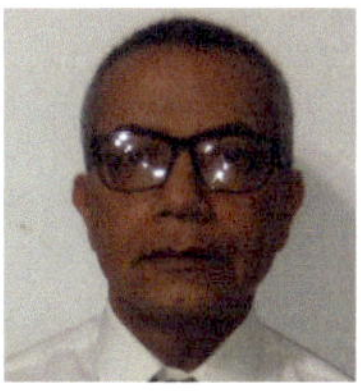

Gilberto Bastidas is a surgeon who graduated from the University of the Andes, Venezuela, with degrees in Pre-hospital Emergency Care, Executive Direction for High Management in Health, and Occupational Health and Safety. He has an MS in Educational Management, an MS in Protozoology, an international master's degree in Public Health and Hospital Management, and a Ph.D. in Parasitology. He is the author of several journal articles and textbooks. He is also a lecturer and a member of the editorial committees of several national and international journals.

Contents

Preface

This book was structured under the documentary research methodology of a narrative type and with the contribution of several authors who have academic prestige and great expertise in the field of zoonosis as a public health problem. It is a useful resource for professionals in the health field and all those interested in the prevention and control of zoonotic diseases.

The chapters that make up this book offer information on the risk factors directly related to zoonotic diseases. They also explain, analyze, and describe concepts related to epidemiological behavior, transmission, pathogenesis, diagnosis, treatment, and prevention and control of these diseases. The book describes the reciprocal positive and negative consequences that arise from the interaction between humans and animals within the biological, social, and cultural context where it develops.

Gilberto Bastidas
Department of Public Health and Institute of Medical
and Biotechnological Research,
Faculty of Health Sciences,
University of Carabobo,
Carabobo, Venezuela

Section 1

Introduction

Chapter 1

Introductory Chapter: Why the Study of Zoonoses?

Gilberto Bastidas

1. Introduction

Zoonoses are infectious diseases that are naturally transmitted between vertebrate animals and humans due to the close interaction between the two, with severe consequences for public health and significant economic losses for both the family and the nation. It is a complex group of pathologies caused by a great diversity of pathogens with diverse biological cycles and modes of dissemination. The health problem is such that zoonoses currently represent about 70% of infectious diseases of man (new and existing) in most countries, with more than 200 known types of these [1].

They are a complex group of diseases caused by a diversity of pathogenic microorganisms with varied biological cycles and modes of dissemination that constitute a real challenge for public health with full validity of their complexity and therefore the need to consider multiple perspectives for the approach, without a doubt, all related to epidemiology, biology, and social sciences; in this sense, it is essential to consider and develop integrated interventions that result from the knowledge of the process that defines zoonosis, objective of this book, that is, to show concepts, theories, and arguments about it that contribute to the understanding of such a complicated phenomenon [1].

2. Reasons for researching and studying zoonosis

At present, it is necessary to provide information to health sciences professionals, health authorities, and the general population on zoonosis; hence, the updating and condensation of the concepts that define this type of disease is imperative. Main objective of this book entitled: "Zoonosis of Public Health Interest," because worldwide there has been an increase in the incidence and prevalence of zoonoses, and even the emergence and re-emergence of some of them are mainly due to the penetration of the human beings in territories with natural reservoirs of infection, climate and environmental change, the development of diagnostic methods with greater sensitivity and specificity, demographic factors such as migration, forced human displacement and population growth, international production and distribution of food, and the deficient sanitary programs destined to the control of these pathologies [2].

The information contained in this book can contribute in each country in the field of primary health systems with the evaluation of the epidemiological and epizootic panorama of the human and animal population as a key element of their epidemiological surveillance systems for the prevention and control of these diseases. These diseases are transmitted between animals and humans; therefore, quality, complete, and current data are provided on different facets or aspects that define the origin, approach, and control of zoonosis as pathologies of great interest to public health because they result from the close relationship between animal and human health, the difficulties that many countries, mainly those with low economic income, have in objectively determining the degree of affectation, and the imbalance caused by zoonotic diseases in the health system, and of course in the quality of life of the individual and the community [3].

This book makes clear the negative implications for public health (due to the high morbidity and mortality) of the relationship in the category of zoonosis between humans and animals, which goes beyond the simple transmission of pathogens, since the zoonosis is a complex process in which various factors converge, from the human sphere, among which epidemiological behavior, space, population, economy, social structure, and cultural order stand out [4]. In this sense, it corresponds to the health professional the interest in reviewing the written works that are produced on zoonoses, particularly due to the great composition that this type of pathology has that compromises animal and human health, and because these diseases are not approached with sufficient depth in the academic training programs of the health sciences sector, which translates into terrible confusion and ignorance about the mechanism of transmission, pathogenesis, diagnosis, treatment, prevention, and control of such fearsome pathologies [5].

This book shows investigations of different variables of zoonosis such as health risk, biological-environmental relationship, treatment, emergence of pathogens, health policies, and basic concepts on the transmission of diseases between animals and humans. Since, in the context of complex reality in which zoonosis moves, it is essential to study the factors that contribute to the current situation of these diseases in the world. So, it is a key to describe them from multiple perspectives, because in this order of ideas it stands out the appearance of new zoonotic diseases and the modification of the form of transmission of some existing ones that do not allow the explanation of the events for their adequate approach and can even generate wrong diagnoses. Hence, the information provided in this book points to the global epidemiological attack and with a comprehensive vision for being the one that ensures greater effectiveness in terms of population coverage and, therefore, in prevention and control [6].

In general terms, the importance of understanding and rigorous attention to the animal-man relationship in the genesis of diseases in the context of public health is described, with particular interest in areas or regions marked by poverty and poor services. Health and other factors on which the need to theoretically base the conceptual elements of zoonosis that are explicitly recorded in this writing is based, can contribute to the scientific planning of health between humans and animals in relation to the constants changes that occur in the dynamics of the transmission [7].

The exposed concepts can serve as tools to increase the response capacity of health systems for the development and implementation of plans and training programs for health personnel, as well as for health education to the population, in general, in terms of zoonosis, and specifically the experiences that are narrated can be used for the timely attention of endemic and epidemic foci for the follow-up of cases and for the implementation of an adequate information and epidemiological surveillance system [8]. In this sense, you are invited to carefully read the theoretical framework presented in this work.

Author details

Gilberto Bastidas
Department of Public Health, Institute of Medical and Biotechnological Research, University of Carabobo, Venezuela

*Address all correspondence to: bastidasprotozoo@hotmail.com

References

[1] World Health Organization (WHO). Zoonosis. 2020. Available from: https://www.who.int/es/news-room/fact-sheets/detail/zoonoses

[2] Pan American Health Organization (PAHO). Guide for epizootiological surveillance. 2002. Available from: http//www.com

[3] Picco N. Rodents as Transmitters of Zoonotic Diseases. Argentina: National University of Rio Cuarto; 2003 Available from: http://newweb.www.paho.org/Spanish/PED/te_rdes.htm

[4] Pan American Health Organization (PAHO). Veterinary public health. Editorial. Bulletin of the Pan American Health Organization. 1992;**113**(5-6):494-501

[5] Fuentes M, Pérez L, Suárez Y, Soca M, Martínez A. Zoonosis as science and its social impact. Veterinary Electronic Journal. 2006;**7**(9):1-19

[6] Bastidas G, Medina T, Bastidas D. Parasitic Diseases in Emergency and Reemergence Environments. Spanish: Spanish Academic Publisher; 2018

[7] Báez F. Zoonosis: A public health problem. Clinical and Social Medicine. 2019;**3**(3):104-105

[8] Bastidas G. Contributions of epidemiology to the control of leishmaniasis. Journal of Public Health of Colombia. 2019;**21**(4):1-4

Section 2

Zoonoses Generalities

Chapter 2

Zoonosis Aspects to Consider for Its Approach

Gilberto Bastidas

Abstract

This paper constitutes a compendium of introductory aspects to consider the approach to zoonosis useful for health sciences professionals. It was based on a documentary review of scientific literature based on a narrative approach. The information found was grouped into the following chapters: the concept of zoonosis, general aspects of zoonosis, an overview of zoonosis in the world, and theoretical and methodological interventions on zoonosis. Finally, and as a contribution from the researchers, conclusions are provided.

Keywords: zoonosis, public health, vertebrate animals, human beings, health programs

1. Introduction

Zoonosis (due to viruses [45%], bacteria [28%], parasites [20%], and fungi [7%]) cause damage to health because they represent 70% of the infectious pathologies that affect human beings and with a significant compromise of animal health (of 1 415 pathogenic agents for humans, 868 zoonosis have been described, and 80% of the latter are capable of affecting different species of animals), which implies a considerable economic burden for the countries, fundamentally derived from their health system [1–3].

In addition, the underreporting of zoonosis in many countries, especially those with low incomes, is notable, among other things, to deficiencies in health promotion and education, poor health coverage, limited hospital and laboratory infrastructure, poor inter-institutional interaction and, especially the application of deficient sanitary control programs [4, 5].

These diseases are often underestimated as a public health problem despite their significant impact on morbidity and mortality (43.6% are distributed throughout the world, of which 63.3% appear in Africa) compared to other pathologies that affect humans and animals [3, 6–9].

Mainly due to the lack of knowledge of the real magnitude of the problem (good records are not kept), the noncompliance in the application of the control programs that already exist in each country, and because of the key concepts that constitute the theoretical framework of zoonoses as an area of knowledge They are scattered in various bibliographic sources, which makes access difficult [3, 6–9].

The objective of the present written is to make a compilation of information on the last point, that is, a concentration and updating of relevant aspects that exist in the world literature on the subject based on a narrative approach. Since solid knowledge is that health professionals can achieve significant achievements in the prevention, control, and eradication of zoonosis [3, 6–9].

2. Methodology

The present work was based on the documentary review of scientific literature in electronic and physical format on aspects of zoonosis based on the systematic analysis and narrative description of what was found, for which virtual databases were used (Bireme/PAHO, Medline, PudMed, and Scielo) from descriptors related to the topic. Repeated documents and those without clear conclusions and without originality were excluded. All original articles published up to December 2021 were included. The relevant ideas were grouped into four aspects that can be read independently, in order to facilitate their review:

1. The concept of zoonosis,

2. General aspects of zoonosis,

3. Overview of zoonosis in the world, and

4. Theoretical and methodological interventions of zoonosis.

Finally, and as a contribution from the researchers, conclusions are provided.

2.1 The concept of zoonosis

This word derives from the Greek roots zoos (animal) gnosis (disease). Its origin is attributed to Rudolf Virchowe, since in the nineteenth century he used this word to refer to diseases shared between man and animals. In 1956 (in the twentieth century) the World Health Organization defined zoonosis as any disease that is naturally transmitted from vertebrate animals to man in a man-centered concept, therefore, three years later this international organism of health reformulates the concept of diseases that are transmitted between animals and man [10, 11].

This last definition of zoonosis is followed by the proposal by Schwalbe, which from the operational-administrative perspective gives it the following meaning: "... those infections and infestations that in nature are shared by man and other lower vertebrate animals" [10–12]. Subsequently, the concepts zoo anthropozoonosis (when the infection is transmitted from animals to humans) and anthropozoonosis (when the infection is transmitted from humans to animals) appear [11, 12].

According to the characteristics of their transmission cycle, zoonosis is classified into (**Table 1**):

In addition, the transmission of a zoonosis between animals and humans can be:

- Direct due to systematic or circumstantial coexistence (they group together a large part of the best-known zoonoses);

Transmission cycle	Type
Direct cycle	Only one vertebrate involved.
Cyclozoonosis	More than one vertebrate is involved.
Metazoonosis	A vertebrate and an invertebrate participate.
Saprozoonosis	Requires an inert element to complete its transmission cycle.
Source: Schwalbe (10), Acha (1986), Bastidas (2018).	

Table 1.
Types of zoonosis according to their transmission cycle.

- Indirect when different elements of the environment, such as soil, water, organic matter, food, and vectors (abundant in etiology and versatile in their form of transmission), intervene;
- Those that can be transmitted directly or indirectly [10, 13, 14].

2.2 General aspects of zoonosis

Due to their form of transmission, zoonosis is divided into:

- Direct (they are transmitted by contact between vertebrate animals and humans, and vice versa), and
- Indirect (includes living or inanimate intermediaries).

They can also be

- Emerging (unknown so far or the result of infection) evolution or modification of pathogenic agents whose pathogenicity, transmitter, or host is known),
- Re-emerging (these are known diseases whose prevalence increases considerably), or
- Exotic (known but never before presented in a certain region).

A disease can be placed in more than one category. In addition, these infections can be:

- Synanthropic (urban cycle) or
- Exoanthropic (sylvatic cycle), and
- Even be mixed [15].

Emerging and re-emerging zoonosis are considered neglected diseases because their prevalence is particularly high in marginalized populations with low incomes without access to health services and where official health institutions neglect to attend to their health needs. In addition, among the conditioning factors of the emergence and re-emergence of zoonosis, demography, ecological and climatic changes, and human behavior are mentioned [16, 17].

2.3 Overview of zoonosis in the world

The key element to describe the epidemiological behavior of zoonosis is the information registry. However, its quality (complete and up-to-date) can be seriously compromised in countries with low economic income, due to poor investment of financial resources and technical difficulties, as well as the frequent political and social conflicts that occur in many of these countries, because private health institutions do not keep records or do so partially or incompletely, and because of the subclinical behavior of some zoonosis that prevents their registration on time [6, 18, 19].

In countries with low economic income, economic support, and the availability of human talent and favorable political will toward the health sector are constantly changing, which has a negative influence on the control and eradication of zoonosis, since they mark periodic cycles of advances and setbacks in the fight with these diseases. Likewise, the scarce or absent intersectoral coordination and the non-perception of zoonosis as an important public health problem by health authorities contribute to the stagnation in the control of these diseases. The need for care and the institutional response to zoonosis control allow it to be grouped into three categories as shown in **Table 2** [6, 20]:

The control and eradication of zoonosis are seriously compromised by a series of factors that ensure their spread, among which are mentioned:

- The ability of some pathogens to infect a wide variety of species,
- The appearance of new zoonosis,
- Immunosuppression of the susceptible (due to chemotherapy, use of steroids, and HIV),
- The tendency of the diseases to remain in a latent or subclinical phase,

Zoonosis	Health action
With significant morbidity and/or mortality	It is present in the epidemiological records. With a sanitary control and epidemiological surveillance program incorporated into the organizational structure of the country's health system. With technical regulations and legal framework. With infrastructure and financing.
Sporadic outbreaks, but in longitudinal follow-up, they are more or less frequent.	With direct or indirect evaluations of its incidence by not necessarily official institutions of the health sector. They lack health control programs.
Rarely therefore its importance for public health is unknown.	They are recorded as isolated and insignificant events, generally by private care services.

Source: Modified from Matamoros [6].

Table 2.
Zoonosis according to its importance, is a health problem.

- The chronic course of many of them,
- The damage to health and the severe economic losses that they produce,
- The complexity of the re-emergence of multiple zoonosis,
- The underestimation of clinical diagnosis and the frequent disarticulation between human and animal health in the approach to zoonosis [21–24].

In addition, the control of zoonosis is affected:

- By not being addressed in a particular way despite the existence of common elements,
- By the constant demographic growth (with greater animal exploitation in an attempt to cover food needs),
- By globalization (with an increase in the displacement of people, animals, and their derivatives),
- Due to the increase in occupational accidents (brucellosis, hepatitis, and tuberculosis, among others),
- Due to climate and ecological change (allows the adaptation of pathogens to new territories),
- Due to the tendency to adopt animals wild as pets, and the resistance of pathogens to the drugs used to combat them (by indiscriminate use) [21–23, 25–27].

In Latin America and the Caribbean, for example, there are 26 priority zoonotic diseases (**Table 3**).

In the world, there are several zoonosis, considered emerging and priority among them are H5N1 and H1N1 influenza, SARS, and most recently Ebola and Zika [28]. Likewise, the stages through which zoonosis goes through to become pandemics are currently described (see **Table 4**).

Strategies to try to predict potential pandemics are also described (**Table 5**).

2.4 Theoretical and methodological interventions for zoonosis

Zoonosis is approached, studied, and intervened by classical or conventional epidemiology through the positivist paradigm that is based on the risk approach in the search for explanations about the health-disease process and about the circumstances that imply damage to human health and animal, due to the economic losses generated by the high figures of morbidity and mortality attributed to zoonotic transmission diseases, which undoubtedly hinder the development of countries [10, 30].

The advances and contributions achieved with the methods and theories of classical epidemiology are great and important, however, for the management of zoonoses, an integral vision is required that allows understanding of the complexity of the relationship between animals and human beings due to ecosystem and intervening social variables since it is necessary to go beyond the mere identification of infectious

Rabies
Leptospirosis
Brucellosis
Tuberculosis
Salmonella
Hydatidosis
Campylobacteria
Escherichia coli
Influenza
Chagas
Leishmaniosis
Venezuelan Equine Encephalitis
Trichinella spiralis
Hantavirus
Plague
Anthrax
Chikungunya
Equine Encephalitis
Dengue
Helminths
Food Borne Illness
Toxoplasmosis
Fasciolosis
Erysipelas
Burkholderia mallei
COVID-19

Source: Drawn from Maxwell [28].

Table 3.
Zoonosis is considered priorities for health authorities in Latin America and the Caribbean.

Pre-emergence (Stage 1): The infectious agent is in its natural reservoir, but the alteration of the transmission dynamics due to environmental, ecological, social, and economic alterations allows:
Expansion within the host population.
The spread to a new region.
It is transmitted to another non-host population.
That reaches the human being.
Large-scale agricultural or demographic changes, such as transport of livestock, to the region where the infectious agent has a niche or movement of wildlife to other regions in search of food, result in multidirectional transmission. For example, transmission like this can be between livestock and non-human primates and that can increase the probability that the pathogen reaches humans and spreads among different populations.
Advance to the second stage??.
Localized emergency (Stage 2): The causative agent spreads from wildlife or livestock to people due to the slaughter of wild animals and from exposure to fomites in markets, on farms, or in the wild. It can affect small human groups orstepthen
become large outbreaks. They can be limited (for example, Ebola virus) or not (for example, Hendra virus)
Full pandemic emergency (Stage 3): Transmission is already sustained from person to person and spread is on a large scale driven by global air travel (HIV/AIDS and severe acute respiratory syndrome, among others) and travel for reservoir and vector trade (West Nile virus). This stage depends on a long chain of transmission, so that it can occur, for this reason, pandemics in stage three are considered rare.

Source: Modified from Stephen [29].

Table 4.
Stages in disease emergence.

Determining the relationship between the species of the pathogenic agent and the host. This is particularly important because the species closely related to each other favor the transmission of the etiological agent, that is, it passes easily from one host to another, however, in living beings human emerging pathogen species can come from closely related or distant hosts. The key to transmission to occur is contact.
The emergence of pathogens can be predicted based on the analysis of phylogenetic relationships. In this sense, it is known that wild pathogens that are more closely related to those that affect humans are more certain to infect people in contrast to those distant. Likewise, the analysis of the phylogenetic relationship allows for determining the pathogenesis.
The potential of emerging pathogens across a wide range of hosts (plasticity), thus, emerging pathogens have the ability to successfully transmit between different host taxa, thus increasing the probability of transmission to humans. Hence, the need for a constant study of these mechanisms in order to establish predictions.
The presence of factors that facilitate the passage of a pathogen between different host species (evolutionary capacity), although these aspects are little known, they are related to the ability to mutate. The understanding of these mechanisms facilitates the explanation of the high capacity for jumping between hosts that some species of pathogens have. High transmission efficiency is often related to the ability of the pathogen to employ new transmission routes, hence, massive or generalized epidemic outbreaks are correlated with high transmission efficiency.
The prediction of ligand-receptor binding requires an understanding of the interactions involved between common elements (already existing) or new ones because the binding at the cellular level between the pathogen and the host cell is the initial and indispensable step (binding to the receptor is necessary but not sufficient condition to ensure infection since other factors are required) and it is usually associated with changes in the tropism of the host's tissues. Despite the fact that there are many technological and scientific advances, only the cellular receptor of a little less than half of the pathogens that affect human beings is known. Highly species-specific receptors are considered as a barrier to infection between pathogens and unusual or new hosts.
The prediction of the transmissibility (virulence) of pathogens to humans is the greatest challenge to face in the study of pandemics since pathogen species that behave benignly in their natural hosts can trigger severe or lethal inflammatory responses in the host. New host coevolution patterns.
Source: Modified from Stephen [29].

Table 5.
Prediction of pandemic potential.

agents, pathogenesis, transmission, control, and treatment, in this sense, the paradigms of complexity and chaos have been used for the study of zoonosis [30–34].

The single and multi-causality approaches to risk are not enough to understand and explain the complex interactions that occur in zoonosis, paradigms are required that go beyond system theories, structural functionalism, the inability to control the pathogenic agent, the articulation of the epidemiological discourse to health policies, the ecosystem approach and the social component (behavior and culture in the relationship between equals, social determinants, and inequities in health), in this sense, a holistic approach to zoonoses (prevents the fragmentation and decontextualization of the health problem by considering it broad and complex) [30, 35–41].

Hence, international health organizations issue general and comprehensive recommendations that contribute to adequate surveillance and response capacity in the event of the emergency and re-emergence of zoonosis (see **Table 6**).

These recommendations seek to prevent, monitor, and control zoonosis to reduce its impact on health, but to achieve this, the joint participation of animal health, human health, and the environmental sector are required.

Recommendations
• Generation of sufficient financial resources that are sustainable over time.
• Multisectoral coordination, fundamentally between animal and human health and the ecological field, all action for the control or eradication of zoonosis must be coordinated.
• Approach strategies adapted to local conditions.
• Introduction of information and communication technologies in order to facilitate the exchange of information between the different sectors and favor the analysis of zoonosis situations and the health management of the problem.
• Adaptation or design of programs for the control of zoonosis based on the scientific knowledge that is constantly produced on the subject.
• Training of health personnel with a multidisciplinary approach for the prevention, diagnosis, and treatment of these diseases.
• Create a network of laboratories for the diagnosis of international zoonosis.
• Promote the participation of the social sciences in addressing zoonosis.
• Surveillance of zoonosis is everyone's task.
• Frontal and direct fight against the practices and behaviors that contribute to the genesis and maintenance of zoonosis as endemic.
• Community participation in decision-making regarding their health and quality of life is essential.
• Promote the idea that zoonosis is a problem for everyone, for countries with low, medium, and high economic income.

Source: Ministry of Health [42].

Table 6.
Recommendations for comprehensive surveillance and adequate response to zoonosis.

3. Conclusions

This writing constitutes a brief but concise compendium on zoonosis that starts from the meaning of the word, goes through its general aspects, through the epidemiological panorama, and finally through the theoretical and methodological interventions that it has been the object of, it can then serve as a tool for health professionals and for the community in general in acquiring knowledge about zoonosis or for updating them in the fight against these diseases because with the information it offers, the dynamics of the factors that condition or determine their emergence can be understood, re-emergence, prevalence, and distribution in the animal and human population.

However, in the field of health control of zoonosis and from what is stated in this paper, it is concluded that the approach to zoonosis requires cross-cutting, multidisciplinary, and inter-institutional health care, in addition to the incorporation of social, cultural, and economic concepts that define the animal-man relationship, as well as the consideration of the circumstances that imply the involuntary contact between both actors (often ignored) as a result of mutual coexistence and the incorporation in the epidemiological surveillance of diseases of this type that have a low frequency of appearance.

Author details

Gilberto Bastidas
Department of Public Health, Institute of Medical and Biotechnological Research of the University of Carabobo, Venezuela

*Address all correspondence to: bastidasprotozoo@hotmail.com

References

[1] Yamada A. Zoonoses. Uirusu. 2004;**54**(1):17-22. DOI: 10.2222/jsv.54.17

[2] Pan American Health Organization (PAHO). Zoonosis and Neglected Diseases: Interventions and Research. http://www.paho.org/panaftosa/index.php?option=com_content&view=article&id=137&Itemid=371

[3] Fuentes M, Pérez L, Suárez Y, Soca M, Martinez A. Zoonosis as science and its social impact. Electronic Journal of Veterinary Medicine. 2006;7(9):1-19

[4] Bastidas G. Malaria by *Plasmodium vivax* and deficiency of glucose-6-phosphate dehydrogenase: The Venezuela Case. Annals of Malaria Research. 2018;**1**(1):1001

[5] Cross A, Baldwin V, Roy S, Essex-Lopresti A, Prior L, Harmer N. Zoonosis under our noses. Microbes and Infection. 2019;**21**(1):10-19. DOI: 10.1016/j.micinf.2018.06.001

[6] Matamoros J, Sanín L, Santillana M. Zoonoses and their social determinants: a perspective to consider in Public Health. Journal of Public Health. 2000;**2**(1):17-35

[7] Bastidas G. Epidemiological characteristics of Leishmaniasis. Annals of Infectious Disease and Epidemiology. 2018;**3**(2):1030

[8] Bastidas G, Malave C, Bastidas D. Parasitism in science fiction movies and its use as a tool for control. Scientific Information Magazine. 2019;**98**(6):721-733

[9] Moutou F. Zoonosis infectieuses: risques liés à la faune sauvage [Infectious zoonosis: Risks linked to wildlife]. The Revue du Praticien. 2019;**69**(3):333-335

[10] Schwalbe C. Veterinary Medicine and Public Health. Mexico: Editorial Novaro; 1969

[11] Martínez-Conde J. Guide of the Head Veterinary Inspector. 2-Epizootiology and Zoonosis. Barcelona: Aedos Veterinary Library; 1975

[12] Concise Veterinary Dictionary. Great Inglaterra: Britain. Oxford University Press; 1988

[13] Acha N, Szyfres B. Zoonoses and Communicable Diseases Common to Man and Animals. 2nd ed. Washington, DC: Pan American Health Organization; 1986

[14] Bastidas G, Bastidas D. Some parasites that affect the skin in the human being: Epidemiological aspects. Journal of Dermatology & Cosmetology. 2018;**2**(6):84-85

[15] Dabanch J. Zoonosis. Chilean Journal of Infectology. 2003;**20** (Suppl. 1):S47-S51. DOI: 10.4067/S0716-10182003020100008

[16] Maurera D, Bastidas G. Clinical and epidemiological characteristics of patients with tuberculosis in Carabobo state, Venezuela. Medical Journal of Uruguay. 2019;**35**(2):105-112

[17] Maurera D, Liccioni E, Bastidas G. Tuberculosis and experiences: A look from phenomenology. Journal of Nursing and Humanities. 2019;**23**(55):67-77

[18] Eastwood K, Massey P, Mor S, Bosward K. Publisher: Unraveling zoonotic diseases in Australia. Australian Journal of General Practice. 2018;**47**(3):85

[19] Bastidas G, Bastidas D, Bastidas-Delgado G. The control of

tropical diseases is the health goal to achieve. Science Journal of Public Health. 2019;**7**(5):163-166

[20] Bastidas G, Malave C, Bastidas D. *Blastocystis* sp update on its parasitic role. Bolivian Medical Gazette. 2019;**42**(2):182-188

[21] Steele J. Veterinary public health: Past success, new opportunities. Preventive Veterinary Medicine. 2008;**86**(3-4):224-243

[22] Flores R. The current situation of the most frequent zoonoses in the world. Medical Gazette of Mexico. 2010;**146**:423-429 https://www.anmm.org.mx/GMM/2010/n6/64_vol_146_n6.pdf

[23] Báez F. Zoonosis: A public health problem. Clinical and Social Medicine. 2019;**3**(3):104-105

[24] Brucker M. Novel viruses, zoonotic infections, and travel health. Nursing for Women's Health. 2020;**24**(2):65-66. DOI: 10.1016/j.nwh.2020.02.002

[25] Sánchez A, Prats-van der Ham M, Tatay-Dualde J, García-Galán A, de la Fe C, Corrales J, et al. Zoonosis and occupational health in the veterinary profession. Spanish Magazine of Public Health. 2018;**3**:92

[26] Huertas P, León E, Tarabla H. Zoonosis and veterinary waste disposal in rural practice. Argentine Journal of Microbiology. 2019;**51**(3):251-254. DOI: 10.1016/j.ram.2018.08.004

[27] Macedo Couto R, Ranzani O, Waldman E. Zoonotic Tuberculosis in Humans: Control, Surveillance, and the One Health Approach. Epidemiologic Reviews. 2019;**41**(1):130-144. DOI: 10.1093/epirev/mxz002

[28] Maxwell M, de Freire Carvalho M, Hoet A, Vigilato M, Pompei J, Cosivi O, et al. Building the road to a regional zoonoses strategy: A survey of zoonoses programmes in the Americas. PLoS One. 2017;**12**(3):e0174175

[29] Stephen S, Mazet JAK, Woolhouse M, Parrish CR, Carroll D, Karesh WB, et al. Prediction and prevention of the next pandemic zoonosis. Lancet. 2012;**380**:1955-1196

[30] Acero-Aguilar M. Zoonoses and other public health problems related to animals: Reflections on their theoretical and methodological approaches. Journal of Health Management and Policies. 2016;**15**(31):232-245

[31] Arch-Tirado E, Javier R-MJ. Sciences of complexity and chaos as tools in the analysis of the proliferation of vectors and zoonosis. Surgery and Surgeons. 2009;**77**:341-350

[32] Abdel K, Hernández D, Hidalgo O, Hidalgo S, Hung F, Lorenzo C, et al. Clinical-epidemiological characteristics and knowledge about American tegumentary leishmaniasis in a population of Carabobo, Venezuela. Peruvian Journal of Health Research. 2020;**4**(1):09-16

[33] Reina J. SARS-CoV-2, a new pandemic zoonosis that threatens the world. Vaccine. 2020;**21**(1):17-22. DOI: 10.1016/j.vacun.2020.03.001

[34] Royce K, Fu F. Mathematically modeling spillovers of an emerging infectious zoonosis with an intermediate host. PLoS One. 2020;**15**(8):e0237780. DOI: 10.1371/journal.pone.0237780

[35] Rosenberg F. Social structure and veterinary epidemiology in Latin America. Bol centro Panamericano Fiebre Aftosa. 1986;**53**:3-23

[36] Quevedo E. The Health-disease Process: Towards a Non-positivist Clinic

and Epidemiology. Bogotá: Pontificia Universidad Javeriana; 1990

[37] Bastidas G. Contributions of epidemiology to the control of leishmaniasis. Journal of Public Health of Colombia. 2019;**21**(4):1

[38] Bastidas G, Medina T, Bastidas D. Parasitic Diseases in Emergency and Reemergence Environments. Spanish: Spanish Academic Publisher; 2018

[39] Saadi A, Antoine-Moussiaux N, Marcotty T, Thys S, Sahibi H. Using qualitative approaches to explore the challenges of integrated programs for zoonosis control in developing countries: Example of hydatidosis control in Morocco. Zoonosis Public Health. 2021;**68**(5):393-401. DOI: 10.1111/zph.12814

[40] Talbot B, Kulkarni M, Colautti R. Convergence research for emerging zoonosis. Trends in Parasitology. 2021;**37**(6):465-467. DOI: 10.1016/j.pt.2021.03.008

[41] Institute of Medicine. Sustaining Global Surveillance and Response to Emerging Zoonotic: Microbial recommendations the United States. Washington, D.C: National Academy Press; 2009

[42] Ministerio de salud y protección social (Minsalud). Estrategia de gestión integral de zoonosis-EGI-zoonosis. 2017. https://www.minsalud.gov.co/sites/rid/Lists/BibliotecaDigital/RIDE/VS/PP/ET/egi-zoonosis-documento-ultimo.pdf

Section 3

Public Health Interest Zoonosis

Chapter 3

Rabies: Incurable Biological Threat

Jitendrakumar Bhogilal Nayak,
Jeetendrakumar Harnathbhai Chaudhary,
Prakrutik Prafulchandra Bhavsar, Pranav Ashok Anjaria,
Manojbhai N. Brahmbhatt and Urvish Pravinbhai Mistry

Abstract

Rabies is a lethal zoonotic disease that affects all the homeotherms, including humans, and is caused by the Rabies virus of *Rhabdoviridae* family. Every year, this disease kills about 55,000 individuals globally. The stray dog is a key player in the spread of rabies. The disease is usually transmitted through the bite of a rabid animal. After being exposed to the virus, the virus must travel to the brain before generating symptoms. Delirium, unusual behaviour, hallucinations, hydrophobia and insomnia may occur as the condition advances. Diagnostic tests such as direct fluorescent antibody test (dFAT), direct rapid immunohistochemical test (dRIT), lateral flow assay (LFA), reverse transcriptase polymerase chain reaction (RT-PCR), nuclear sequencing, etc. are used in diagnosis of this dreadful disease. The genotype and lineage of the rabies virus can be determined via N gene sequencing and phylogenetic analysis. There is no effective treatment for rabies. Even though a tiny number of people have survived rabies, the disease is usually fatal. Rabies can be completely avoided in people if they receive timely and adequate medical treatment. Vaccinating and sterilising the dogs in our neighbourhoods effectively and humanely limit their population and eliminate rabies in both dogs and humans.

Keywords: dFAT, N gene, rabies, street virus, vaccine

1. Introduction

Rabies is a highly fatal viral infection of the central nervous system caused by the Rabies virus, which belongs to the genus Lyssavirus of the *Rhabdoviridae* family that affects all warm-blooded animals and is a major occupational anthropozoonosis. It is one of the oldest recognised diseases. The word rabies comes from the Latin word *rabere*, which meant to be insane, enraged or ravenous. It is one of numerous zoonotic diseases that go unnoticed, resulting in more than 55,000 deaths per year. According to the Association for Prevention and Control of Rabies in India (APCRI) in 2003, a person dies of rabies every 9 minutes. It is one of the most important zoonotic diseases in history, with a fatality rate of around 100% and a global distribution [1, 2]. While rabies is thought to affect all mammalian species, including nonhuman primates and humans, it is not predominantly a human disease. Human infection is an unintended consequence of the disease's reservoir in wild and domestic animals. In the natural world, rabies is a disease that affects wild carnivores, with reservoirs and vectors including dogs, cats, wolves, foxes, coyotes, jackals, raccoons, skunks and bats. Bats are the main tanks for 10 known lyssavirus serotypes [3]. In 400 BC, Aristotle stated that 'dogs suffer from the madness. This causes them to become very irritable and all animals they bite become diseased'.

Rabies is sustained in two epidemiological cycles, one urban and the other sylvatic. Dogs are the principal reservoir host in the urban rabies cycle. This cycle is most prevalent in areas of Africa, Asia, Central and South America where there are a large number of unvaccinated, semi-owned or stray dogs. In Europe and North America, the sylvatic (or wildlife) cycle is the most common. In animals, disease patterns might be relatively stable or evolve into a slow-moving epidemic.

The skin or mucous membrane is the most common site of rabies virus entrance in humans and animals, where the virus enters the muscle and subcutaneous tissue through biting, licking or scratching by a rabies-virus-infected animal. Acute encephalomyelitis is the pathogenic manifestation in the CNS. In animals, disease can manifest itself in two ways. The classical or encephalitic (furious) form of rabies accounts for 80–85% of rabies cases. Hydrophobia, pharyngeal spasms and hyperactivity are all symptoms of the furious type of rabies, which can lead to paralysis, coma and death. The dumb type, also known as the paralytic form, is characterised by the development of pronounced and flaccid muscular weakness and is less prevalent. In humans, symptoms of cerebral dysfunction, agitation, anxiety and confusion develop. Later the person experiences abnormal behaviour, delirium, hallucinations, insomnia and respiratory failure. Once the symptoms develop, the disease is often fatal.

Even though Louis Pasteur achieved his first breakthrough against rabies with post-exposure vaccination in 1885, the disease continues to haunt the mankind, particularly in impoverished countries, more than 125 years later [4]. Despite recent advances in diagnosis, post-exposure treatment, the production of human and veterinary vaccines and the control of rabies in dogs and wild animals, rabies remains a major health hazard in many countries in Africa, South America and Asia and an economic burden for both developed and developing countries. Rabies is currently found on all continents except Antarctica, although Asia and Africa account for more than 95% of human mortality. Domestic/wild animals, as well as humans, are the primary transmitters. Many countries, including Japan, the United Kingdom, Denmark, Sweden, Greece, Scandinavia, Iceland, Portugal, New Zealand and Australia, are rabies-free, according to the World Health Organisation (WHO). Vaccination, public awareness, responsible participation, continued cooperation among stakeholders and the removal of the stray dog population are some of the measures to avoid rabies [5].

2. History

The deity of death was accompanied by a dog as the ambassador of death in India about 3000 BC. Rabid canines continue to kill 20,000 people each year in modern-day India. The Mosaic Esmuna Code of Babylon, written around 2300 BC, is the first documented record of rabies causing death in dogs and humans. Babylonians had to pay a fine if their dog communicated rabies to another person. Democritus, in the fifth century BC, accurately described the disease in dogs, as did Aristotle in the third century BC [6].

The medical literature of the ancient world was littered with ineffective folk cures. Scribonius Largus, a physician, proposed a poultice of cloth and hyena skin, while Antaeus suggested a concoction prepared from a hung man's skull. The Roman scholar Celsus correctly predicted that rabies was transmitted through the saliva of the bitten animal in the first century A.D. He wrongly suggested that placing the victim under water would cure rabies. Those who did not drown succumbed to rabies. In eighteenth-century America, the most intriguing rabies therapy was the usage of madstones. Madstones are calcified hairballs found in ruminant stomachs including cows, goats and deer. They were supposed to have healing properties since they drew the craziness from the bite wound.

In the 1880s, the first effective rabies treatment was developed. When Louis Pasteur, a French chemistry instructor, was experimenting with chicken cholera, he discovered that virulent cultures exposed to the elements no longer caused sickness. He also discovered that chickens inoculated with this weaker or 'attenuated strain' were immune to fresh, virulent cultures. Pasteur then attempted an attenuated anthrax vaccination in cattle. It was successful! He next turned his attention to the world's scourge, rabies. Pasteur wanted more time to purify his attenuated vaccine before trying it on himself, despite the positive results of his initial animal experiments. In the year 1885, a rabid dog mauled a 9-year-old kid named Joseph Meister. The wounds were treated by a local doctor, who informed Joseph's family that Louis Pasteur was the only person who could rescue him. Pasteur consented only after speaking with a few of genuine doctors, who stated Joseph was a 'dead lad walking'. Joseph recovered completely after receiving 13 inoculations in just 11 days. The nerve tissue vaccine developed by Louis Pasteur in 1885 was a success, and it was modified over time to decrease the typical severe side effects [7].

3. Mode of transmission

Although dogs are the predominant reservoirs, other domesticated animals and wildlife also play a role in rabies transmission [8]. The virus can easily be passed from one mammal to another, whether they are of the same species or not. Humans are most infected with rabies after being bitten or scratched by an infected dog or cat. Bats, foxes, coyotes, skunks, raccoons, wolves, opossums and other animals are among the commonly infected wild or feral animals. Rabid dogs infect most people in poor countries. These dogs are frequently aggressive and drool frequently, although they act very withdrawn. Humans and domestic animals contract the disease after coming into contact with infected saliva.

Bites, non-bite exposure and human-to-human transmission are all possible routes for rabies transmission. The most common way to contract rabies is through a bite from a rabid animal, although infection can also be spread through skin wounds contaminated by infected saliva. The incubation period is the time between the bite and the onset of symptoms, and it can span anywhere from weeks to months. Because the virus has not yet made it to the saliva, a bite by the animal during the incubation stage carries no danger of rabies. Other inoculation routes are uncommon. The rabies virus can enter the body through wounds or direct contact with mucous membranes. The virus cannot pass through intact skin. The chance of contracting rabies from a bite (5–80%) is at least 50 times higher than the risk of contracting it from a scratch (0.1–1%). Virus particles are present in all the body secretions 2 days after it first enters the CNS, and the victim is fully contagious. At or shortly after this point, clinical symptoms develop.

Non-bite exposures are uncommon sources of transmission. Non-bite exposure includes scratches, abrasions, open wounds or mucous membranes infected with saliva or materials such as rabid animal brain tissue. Inhalation of aerosolised rabies virus is another non-bite route of infection, although most people, except for laboratory personnel, are unlikely to encounter an aerosolised rabies virus. Rare cases of rabies in humans have been reported because of breathing air in a cave home to thousands of bats. As rabies virus can be found in the milk of infected animals, milk can be a vehicle for virus transmission. During the consumption of infected milk, an ulcer, abscess or other lesion in the mouth may trigger rabies. Transmission between humans is extremely rare, although it can happen through transplant surgery or even more rarely through bites, kisses or sexual relations. There were outlined a number of cases of rabies transmission from human to human through cornea transplant. Some dogs slaughtered for human consumption may be infected with the rabies virus, exposing handlers of dog meat to the disease because the virus may be present in the meat's nerves. Rabies transmission to butchers is increased during handling, catching, loading, transportation and holding prior to slaughter.

4. Pathogenesis

The virus enters the body via transdermal inoculation (wounds) or direct contact with infectious materials (saliva, cerebrospinal fluid, nerve tissue) on mucous membranes or skin lesions. The virus is incapable of penetrating intact skin. After its entry in the skin, it can undergo eclipse phase, which is not easily detected. Virus replication begins in non-nervous tissue such as striated muscle cells at the site during this phase [9]. The virus can survive for a long time here, influencing the incubation period (the time between exposure and the development of sickness) in different individuals. The virus uses nicotinic acetylcholine receptors to connect to the cells at the inoculation site. The amount of virus acquired through the bite, the amount of tissue innervated and the tissue's proximity to the brain all influence how long it takes for clinical indications to appear. The faster the signals appear, the higher the dose and the closer it is to the central nervous system. It can last anywhere from 4 days to several years, but it usually lasts between 20 and 90 days. Muscle cell replication occurs without causing any noticeable signs. It normally does not elicit an immunological response at this time, but if antibodies are present, it can be neutralised. Because the virus is neurotropic, its absorption into peripheral neurons is critical for infection progression. The neuromuscular spindles are a critical entrance point for viruses into the neurological system. Motor end plates can also be used to gain access to the nervous system by the virus [9].

The rabies virus can infect a variety of cell types, although it is most seen in neurons. Virus infection and replication include several processes, including:

1. Adsorption: It is the process of fusing the rabies virus envelope to the host cell membrane, which may entail contact with the G protein and certain cell surface receptors.

2. Penetration: Infection of the host cell by the virus by pinocytosis (via clathrin-coated pits).

3. Uncoating: Virions clump together in large endosomes (cytoplasmic vesicles), and viral membranes merge with endosomal membranes, which results in uncoating which exposes the virus's genetic content.

4. Transcription: *Rhabdoviridae* are negative-stranded RNA viruses that need the utilisation of an RNA polymerase (L gene) enzyme to convert the negative-stranded mRNA segment to a positive-stranded segment before translation.

5. mRNA: RNA that acts as a template for the synthesis of proteins.

6. Translation: The process of converting the mRNA code into N, P, M, G and L proteins.

7. Replication: In the host cell, the virus genetic material is amplified.

8. Assembly: Virus components are assembled. The ribonucleoprotein (RNP) core is formed by the N–P–L complex encasing negative-stranded genomic RNA, while the M protein forms a capsule, or matrix, surrounding the RNP.

9. Budding: The completed virus buds from the M–RNP complex's interaction with the glycoprotein in the plasma membrane.

After replication in the originating neuron's cell body, infection spreads through multiple neurons by retrograde axonal transport and transsynaptic dissemination. The ability of a virus to proliferate within the CNS via synaptic connections is known as transsynaptic spread. The rabies virus infects neurons, causing changes in neurotransmitter function that impact serotonin, GABA and muscarinic acetylcholine transmission. After that, acinar cells are infected, and the virus is discharged into the oral cavity. This explains why the virus can be found in saliva.

5. Pathology

In rabies, there are no visible lesions. Rabies lesions are microscopic, restricted to the CNS and have a wide range of severity. Except for early necrosis of neurons with cytoplasmic inclusion bodies in the afflicted nerve cells, they may be difficult to detect. Pathologic evidence of rabies encephalomyelitis (inflammation) in brain tissue and meninges includes the following:

1. Mononuclear infiltration

2. Perivascular cuffing of lymphocytes or polymorphonuclear cells

3. Lymphocytic foci

4. Babes nodules consisting of glial cells

5. Negri bodies

There are diffuse perivascular cuffing, neuronophagic nodules and other alterations for neuron destruction throughout the brain in some cases. The hippocampus in the brain stem and the gasserian ganglia are notably affected. Lesions in the gasserian ganglia are more particular, occur earlier and are more consistent than lesions in other parts of the body. Babes nodules, which are clumps of growing glial cells, are the major lesion. Most of the histopathologic markers of rabies were identified by 1903, but rabies inclusions had yet to be discovered. Dr. Adelchi Negri reported the discovery of the Negri body, which he believed to be the etiologic agent of rabies. Negri bodies are round or oval inclusions within the cytoplasm of nerve cells of rabies-infected animals. The size of Negri bodies can range from 0.25 to 0.27 metres. The pyramidal cells of Ammon's horn and the Purkinje cells of the cerebellum are the most potential sites for them. They're also found in medulla cells and a variety of other ganglia. Negri bodies can be detected in the salivary glands, tongue and other organs' neurons. They're generally found in the hippocampus in dogs, but they are more common in the Purkinje cell of the cerebellum in cattle. In preparations stained with Mann's or Seller's stain, a granular, somewhat basophilic interior structure can be detected. When the virus infects the salivary glands centrifugally, the acinar epithelium undergoes degenerative alterations that lead to necrosis, primarily affecting the mucogenic cells of the mandibular salivary glands. Fluorescent antibody methods and electron microscopy can easily show virus within these cells. The degenerative alterations are accompanied by a moderate infiltration of lymphocytes and plasma cells.

6. Clinical signs

Rabies clinical indications are rarely conclusive. Rabid animals of all species show similar symptoms of CNS abnormalities, with slight differences across species. It's likely that the animal is seeking solitude. Rabid wild animals may lose their fear of humans, and traditionally nocturnal species may be found walking around during the day. The clinical course can be split into three stages: prodromal, furious and dumb.

Prodromal form—The term prodromal is initial period of rabies with non-specific period.

Furious form—It refers to animals in which the aggression is pronounced.

Dumb form—It refers to animals in which the behavioural changes are minimal, and the disease is manifest principally by paralysis.

6.1 Prodromal form

It is initiated when rabies virus travels up the peripheral nerve axons to the spinal ganglia which form the junction between the peripheral and central nervous systems.

6.2 Furious form

During this stage, there is very little evidence of paralysis. The animal becomes restless and may lash out with its fangs, claws, horns or hooves at the slightest provocation. These animals lose their fear of other animals and lose their caution. Carnivores infected with this strain of rabies are known to roam freely, attacking other animals, including humans and moving objects. Rabid dogs may shatter their teeth by chewing the wire and frame of their cages. Saliva either flows out of the mouth or is churned into a foam that can stick to the lip and face. Progressive paralysis leads to death.

6.3 Paralytic form

The paralysis of the throat and masseter muscles is the initial symptom, which is typically accompanied by excessive salivation and the inability to swallow. Dogs tend to drop their lower jaw. These animals aren't violent and only bite occasionally. The paralysis spreads quickly to all regions of the body and may lead to coma, and many die within a few hours.

7. Variations in signs and symptoms in different species

7.1 Cattle

Incubation takes about 3 weeks on average, although it can take anywhere from a few weeks to several months. Early indications of paralysis include knuckling of the hind fetlocks, sagging and swaying of the hindquarters while walking and typical deviation or flaccidity of the tail to one side. In this species, yawning is a common phenomenon. Soon after yawning, the animal begins to bellow, which continues until it reaches paralysis. One of the most common symptoms is saliva drooling. The penis of bulls in this stage is paralysed. Animals may attack other animals or inanimate objects with ferocity. Lactation in dairy cows ends abruptly. Sexual arousal is common. These symptoms linger during 24–48 hours, after which the animal collapses in a paralysed state and dies within a few weeks.

7.2 Sheep

The signs are comparable to those of cattle. Sexual arousal, attacks on humans or each other and intense wool pulling have all been observed. There are twitches in the muscles, and salivation is observed. There is no excessive bleating. Most sheep are quiet and anorectic.

7.3 Goat

Aggressive and continuous bleating seen.

7.4 Pigs

Excitement, a tendency to strike, dullness and incoordination are some of the indications that have been identified. There is nasal twitching, quick chewing movements, profuse salivation and clonic convulsions.

7.5 Horses

Show signals of anguish and agitation on a regular basis. These indications are frequently accompanied by rolling. They can bite or strike with ferocity. Abnormal postures, frequent whining, kicking, biting, colic and abrupt onset of lameness in limbs followed by recumbency are all the symptoms. Paddling convulsions and ultimate paralysis are followed by sternal and lateral recumbency.

7.6 Cats

The symptoms are identical to those seen in dogs. Two to four days after the initial symptoms start, the posterior part of the body is paralysed.

8. Clinical signs in humans

Incubation, prodromal stage, acute neurological phase, coma and death are the five stages of clinical manifestations.

8.1 Incubation phase

It takes 30–90 days for rabies to develop, although it can take anything from 5 days to more than 2 years after initial exposure. It may be slightly shorter in children and vary depending on the bite place.

8.2 Prodromal phase

During this period, the first signs and symptoms appear. Some of the symptoms include fever, fatigue, sore throat, cough, dyspnea, anorexia, dysphagia, nausea, vomiting, abdominal pain, diarrhoea, headache, vertigo, anxiety, irritability and anxiousness. Agitation, photophobia, priapism, increased libido, sleeplessness and depression are all symptoms that could indicate encephalitis, psychiatric problems or brain conditions.

8.3 Acute neurologic period

This stage starts with symptoms of central nervous system dysfunction, such as anxiety, insomnia, disorientation, agitation, strange behaviour, paranoia, terror and hallucinations and progresses to delirium. During the later stages, significant amount of saliva is produced together with an inability to swallow, resulting in hydrophobia due to paralysed throat and jaw. If hyperactivity is present, the condition is classed as furious, and if paralysis is present, the disease is categorised as dumb. Periods of rapid, uneven breathing may begin near the end of this phase, followed by coma and death.

9. The virus and its genome

Rabies virus is a single-stranded, negative-sense, unsegmented, enveloped RNA virus with a rod or bullet shape. Five proteins are encoded by the viral genome. In the cytoplasm of infected cells, viral RNA uncoils. A virion-associated RNA-dependent RNA polymerase transcribes the genome. Individual viral proteins are subsequently translated from viral RNA. The creation of progeny negative-stranded RNA begins with the synthesis of positive-stranded RNA templates [10]. The RNA is responsible for coding five genes: *N*, Nucleoprotein, 1424 bp; *P*, Transcriptase associated, 991 bp;*M*, Matrix, 805 bp; *G*, Glycoprotein, 1675 bp and *L*, Transcriptase, 6475 bp while one pseudogene intron of approximately 700 bp makes total genome size of $\approx$ 12Kb. *N* gene is responsible for the nucleic acid, so it holds more importance for the diagnostic and evolutionary tracking of the disease.

9.1 Important strains of the virus

Pasteur—Pasteur passaged the virulent 'street' virus of rabies in the rabbit by intracranial inoculation. After several passages in the rabbit, virus has modified several characteristics and started giving similar kind of only paralytic forms in rabies and similar incubation period and without producing intracytoplasmic Negri bodies. The virus is also identified as the 'fixed' virus. The virus is used to produce vaccine.

CVS—International bodies have approved and recommended a variety of vaccine strains for rabies vaccine production around the world. The rabies challenge virus standard (CVS-11) strain is one of these strains that has been licenced for vaccine manufacturing, is recommended for use in (Rapid Fluorescent Foci Inhibition Test) RFFIT and is utilised as a challenge virus around the world. It is a well-characterised strain that was adapted in mice from the original Pasteur rabies virus discovered in 1882.

9.2 Difference in the street and fixed viruses

Street virus	Fixed virus
Isolated from infected animal or human	Isolated from several intracranial passages from rabbits
Causes several encephalopathies after varying incubation period	Less infective but cause disease after a fixed incubation of 7–10 days
Negri bodies can be demonstrated	Negri bodies are not produced
Not utilised for vaccine production	Suitable and utilised for the vaccine production

10. Need of the genetic study of the virus

A case of human rabies is described in Siberia's polar region by Kuzmin [11] In the year 1999. The victim had been bitten by a wolf. Monoclonal antibodies revealed that the isolate was from arctic fox virus strain. This finding reaffirmed the importance of strain typing rabies virus isolates in areas where it has not yet been done: such characterisation is important for identifying the reservoir host, learning about the virus's natural history in the reservoir and planning future surveillance, post-exposure treatment and public education in the area.

11. Epidemiology of rabies

Epidemiology is the study of distribution and the determinants of the disease. For the better understanding of the topic, epidemiology is given in two separate sections.

11.1 Distribution of the disease

Rabies is found everywhere across the planet, except for islands. Except for Australia and Antarctica, rabies is endemic in many of the countries. Bahrain, Cyprus, Hong Kong, Japan, Malaysia, Maldives, Qatar, Singapore, Lakshdweep, India's Andaman and Nicobar Islands and Timor-Leste are among the Asian countries free of rabies. Antigua and Barbuda, the Bahamas, Barbados, Belize, Falkland Islands,

Jamaica, Saint Kitts and Nevis, Trinidad and Tobago, Uruguay of the Americas subcontinent, and Albania, F.Y.R. of Macedonia, Finland, Gibraltar, Greece, Iceland, Isle of Man, Malta, Portugal, Norway (except Svalbard), United Kingdom and Spain (except Melilla and Ceuta) have all been declared rabies-free. Cape Verde, Congo, Libya, Mauritius, Reunion and Seychelles are the only African countries free of rabies. Fiji, Cook Islands, Vanuatu, Guam, French Polynesia, New Zealand, New Caledonia, Solomon Islands and Papua New Guinea are among the Oceana group of islands that are rabies-free [12, 13]. Bangladesh and India are the most affected, followed by Nepal, Myanmar, Bhutan, Thailand and Indonesia. Nepal is one of the countries in the world with the highest number of human rabies deaths [12, 13].

11.2 Determinants of the disease

Rabies is a unique disease as it can contract a wide range of all the warm-blooded hosts.

11.2.1 Age

Children lack fundamental ethology understanding about dogs, children are more vulnerable to the sickness and animal bites. When children disturb dogs while they are feeding, resting, mating or terrified, dogs get violent and bite them. According to research, the disease claimed the lives of 37% of children aged 5–14. [14]. Although the people from all the age groups are susceptible to the disease. The common site of bite in case of children is the face, and often children tend to hide the animal bite marks due to fear of scolds from the parents [15].

11.2.2 Gender

Males are more prone to contract to the disease as they are usually accessed to go out of the homes for earning or playing. In a study it was found that the ratio of men to women suffering from the disease was 4:1 [16].

11.2.3 Area

Awareness plays a major role in the succession of the disease. In urbanised area, availability of the medical facilities and awareness is a factor which may show reduced cases of the disease contrary; in rural areas, many socio-economic and religious factors are responsible for the disease spread as in many part of Gujarat, India, there are temples of 'Hadkai mata', mythologically protecting the people bitten by dogs from the rabies. The bite of a rabies-infected dog causes over 95% of human cases, which disproportionately afflict rural people, particularly children, in economically challenged countries of Africa and Asia [17].

11.2.4 Dog population

Majority of the rabies cases are occurring in the Southeast Asia and that too from the dogs. More the dogs are the factors significantly contributing to the spread of the disease. Stray dogs are generally naive towards the disease while only scanty dogs are vaccinated against the disease. The unvaccinated stray dog population is the biggest factor for the spread of the disease. At least 70% vaccination in the canine population will be taking care of spread of the disease in the animal population [18].

11.2.5 Type of the exposure

11.2.5.1 Animal bite exposure

The disease occurs in two phases. First phase of the disease occurs once rabid dog bites any animal or human. The live viruses travel from the site of the bite to the brain in centripetal manner. The second phase starts when the virus after reaching the brain starts travelling from the brain to the peripheral nerves and induces the clinical signs. The course of the occurrence is directly related to the site of bite. If the site is nearer to the head, disease progression is rapid.

11.2.5.2 Non-bite exposure

The rabies virus is spread by direct contact with saliva or brain/nervous system tissue from an infected animal (such as through broken skin or mucous membranes in the eyes, nose or mouth). Aside from bites and scrapes, there aren't many injuries. One non-bite form of exposure is inhalation of aerosolised rabies virus, although most people, except for laboratory personnel, will not meet an aerosol of rabies virus. Rabies has been transmitted through corneal and solid organ transplants, but these cases are extremely rare [19].

11.2.6 Host susceptibility range

Although all warm-blooded animals are susceptible to rabies and can transmit the RABV, there is significant interspecies heterogeneity in the ability of mammals to act as reservoirs. Rabies is mostly spread by carnivores all over the world [12]. Main cause for the transmission of the virus is wildlife or stray animals, lesser than 10% cases are reported from the domesticated animals such as dogs or cats [20]. Equine and bovine are generally susceptible to the disease, but they are considered as the dead end hosts as they generally do not transmit the disease [21].

There are two types of epidemiological cycle for the occurrence of the disease. Urban and Sylvatic cycles, both the cycles are overlapping to each other and interrelated. Dog, cat, fox, raccoon, jackal, wolf, badger, etc. are the reservoir of the disease while bats are the vector of the disease. In Asian subcontinent, majority of the cases are dog-mediated rabies while in American and European countries, bat-mediated rabies is seen [12]. In India, there are some factors which promote the growth of the stray dogs.

1. Mythologically dogs are related to 'Kal Bhairav', a god of Hinduism, and so from almost all the homes, last feed is offered to the dogs, which helps in the maintenance of the dog population.

2. Vulture population is getting declined day by day which is competitive exclusion parameter for dog food.

3. Open slaughter policies are providing food for sustainability to the dogs outdoor.

4. Open garbage disposal attracts dogs, and many a times they can be utilised as a source to the feed.

12. Diagnosis of rabies

Accurate and timely diagnosis is very important for proper management of the post-exposure prophylaxis and application of the public health control efforts. The disease is diagnosed using a variety of techniques. However, adequate proper collection and submission of post-mortem materials, particularly brain tissues from animals suspected of having rabies, can provide basis for rabies confirmatory diagnosis [22]. Rabies can be difficult to diagnose because, in the early stages, it is easily confused with other diseases or even with a simple aggressive temperament. The reference method for diagnosing rabies is the fluorescent antibody test (FAT), an immunohistochemistry procedure, which is recommended by the World Health Organisation (WHO).

Primary diagnostic methods, such as the direct fluorescent antibody (DFA) test, the direct rapid immunohistochemistry test (dRIT) or pan-lyssavirus polymerase chain reaction (PCR) assays, are used to identify agents. If a proper conjugate or primer/probe is employed, the DFA test, dRIT and PCR offer an accurate diagnosis in 98–100% of cases for all lyssavirus strains. In highly equipped facilities, conventional and real-time PCR may produce speedy results for a large number of samples. Histological procedures such as Seller staining (Negri bodies) are no longer suggested for diagnosis. In the incidence that main diagnostic tests (DFA test, dRIT or pan-Lyssavirus PCR) give unsatisfactory findings, further confirmatory testing (molecular tests, cell culture or mice inoculation tests) on the same sample or repeat primary diagnostic tests on different samples are recommended. Virus isolation in cell culture should be used instead of mice inoculation testing whenever possible. In specialised laboratories, the agent can be characterised utilising monoclonal antibodies, partial and whole genome sequencing and phylogenetic analyses. These approaches can tell the difference between field and vaccine strains, as well as the geographical origin of the field strains. These extremely sensitive tests should only be performed and evaluated by highly experienced experts.

Pre-exposure vaccination and boosters are necessary for all persons and laboratory workers engaged in the management of rabies suspected cases. These individuals are at risk of contracting rabies in a variety of ways. As a result, personal protection equipment (PPE) must be always worn, beginning with the necropsy procedure.

12.1 Identification of the agent

Because the rabies virus inactivates quickly, the specimens should be delivered on ice to the laboratory as soon as possible. Various approaches are used to diagnose rabies, with a focus on brain tissue, although other organs such as salivary glands are also used. Both the cerebellum and the brain stem are recommended for laboratory testing since the virus will be abundant in them and will help in laboratory detection. These portions of the brain can be acquired when the complete brain is removed during necropsy using the skull open approach.

12.2 Collection of samples

The virus can be found in the brain, spinal cord, saliva and salivary glands of a rabies-infected animal. B rain tissue is the preferred specimen for rabies diagnosis, the animal suspected of having rabies should be euthanised in such a way that the brain is not damaged. Only vaccinated and well-trained veterinarians or animal control personnel should remove the animal heads.

Brain sample collection for the accurate diagnosis of rabies is very difficult work and that can be dangerous in the field or if the person is not properly trained. The occipital foramen route of brain sampling is an alternative way of collecting brain samples that does not need open the skull.

12.3 Brain sample collection through the occipital foramen

The brain sample is collected through the occipital foramen by inserting a 5 mm drinking straw or a disposable plastic pipette with a capacity of about 2 mL or by inserting an artificial insemination sheath about 10 cm long into the foramen in the direction of the eye. Brain stem and cerebellum samples can be obtained through the juice straw or artificial insemination sheath (**Figure 1**). This technique of collection should be user-friendly, quick and risk-free for reliable rabies diagnosis [22]. This technique speeds up the more number of brain samples collection simultaneously.

12.4 Animal rabies diagnosis

Laboratory procedures for diagnosing rabies were developed as early as 1800 BC. Adelchi Negri discovered the Negri bodies in 1903, and their diagnostic significance was proved by his wife Lina Negri-Luzzani in 1913 [22]. This cleared the way for the development of a multiplicity of laboratory procedures for rabies confirmation, which are described in the WHO book 'Laboratory Techniques in Rabies' [23] as well as the 'OIE Manual of Diagnostic Tests and Vaccines for Terrestrial Animals' [24].

12.5 Sellar's staining under direct microscopy

Seller's staining method is a quick and easy test. It is a histological test used on brain impressions to show the unique cell lesions known as 'Negri bodies'. These are viral particle aggregates visible as intracytoplasmic inclusion bodies ranging in size from 3 to 30 m in infected neural cells. The Negri bodies are round or oval structures that include basophilic granules in an eosinophilic matrix. This technique has relatively poor sensitivity for the diagnosis of rabies, that's why nowadays this test is no longer recommended [23].

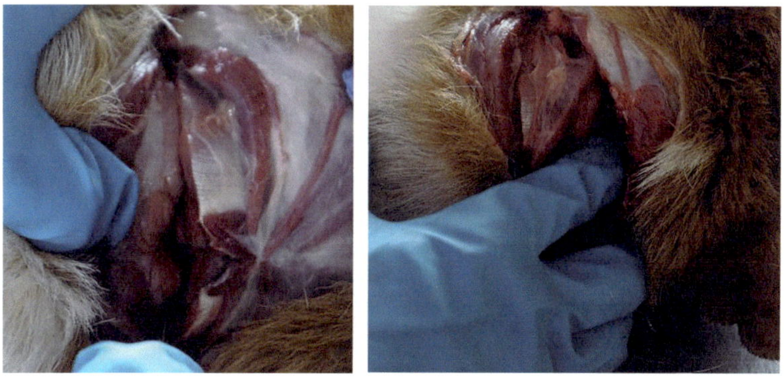

Figure 1.
Brainstem collection through the foramen magnum technique in a dog (captured by the authors).

12.6 Direct fluorescent antibody assay (DFA)

The World Health Organisation (WHO) and the World Organisation for Animal Health (OIE) both endorse the direct fluorescent antibody assay as the most extensively used test for post-mortem confirming diagnosis of rabies. Goldwasser and Kissling created this gold standard test in 1958. The 'Nucleoprotein antigen' (N) of the rabies virus is shown here to be present in fresh brain impressions of rabies suspect animals (**Figure 2**). Such rabies viral inclusions do not exist in the brain impressions of non-rabid animals (**Figure 3**). Furthermore, in a normal laboratory, the DFA has a specificity and sensitivity of about 99% [22].

The DFA is accurate and sensitive. The sensitivity of this test is determined by the quality of the sample (how carefully the brain is sampled as well as the degree of autolysis), the type of lyssavirus and the diagnostic staff's expertise. Impressions are obtained from a composite sample of brain tissue that includes the brainstem. It is air-dried before being immersed in 100% high-grade cold acetone for 1 hour to set the impressions. The impression is withdrawn from the acetone, air-dried and stained with a drop of the appropriate conjugate.

The impression is then incubated for 60 minutes at 37°C. Anti-rabies fluorescent conjugates are commercially available as polyclonal or monoclonal antibodies (MAbs)

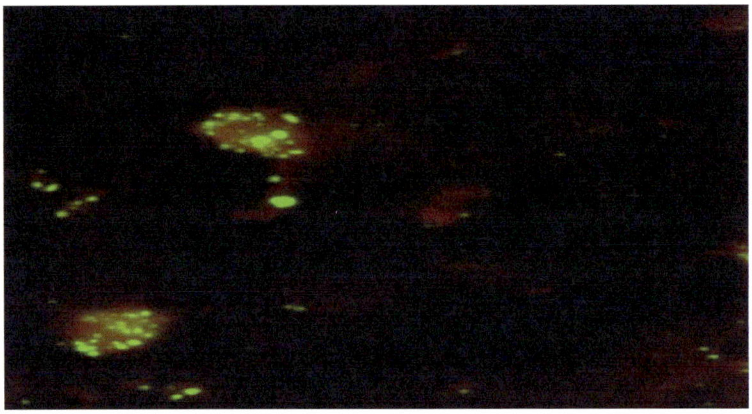

Figure 2.
Rabid animal brain impression, counterstained with Evan's blue and stained with rabies virus antinucleocapsid IgG-FITC conjugate (rabies DFA III, light diagnostics, cat # 6500, captured by authors).

Figure 3.
Non-rabid animal brain impression stained with rabies virus anti-nucleocapsid IgG-FITC conjugate (rabies DFA III, light diagnostics, cat # 6500, captured by authors).

that are specific to whole virus or the N protein of the rabies virus and have been conjugated to the fluorescing dye, fluorescein isothiocyanate (FITC). The DFA slides should be inspected under a fluorescent microscope with a filter that corresponds to the wavelength of the fluorescent conjugate employed. FITC, which is stimulated at 490 nm and re-emits at 510 nm, is the most often used fluorescent dye. The presence of nucleocapsid protein aggregates can be seen by the fluorescence of associated conjugate in an apple green colour. When fresh brain tissue is used, this test is reliable. Bacterial contamination of partially decomposed brains causes nonspecific fluorescence that is difficult to differentiate from specific fluorescence owing to N antigen, making it inappropriate for this test.

12.7 Direct rapid immunohistochemistry test (dRIT)

The Centers for Disease Control and Prevention (CDC) in Atlanta, Georgia, developed dRIT, which is one of the most important breakthroughs in the diagnosis of Rabies. This test also detects the N protein of the rabies virus in rabies brain impressions. A suspected animal brain smear is fixed with buffered formalin before being processed further. Following appropriate viral fixation, the antigen was treated with a biotinylated monoclonal antibody cocktail that was highly concentrated and purified (to N protein). After that, an indicator and streptavidin peroxidase are added. The aggregation of viral clusters is seen as brick red clusters within the cell, along the axons and throughout the brain impression (**Figure 4**). Negative brain impressions show no such brick red inclusions.

This 1-hour test method is helpful in field conditions since the results may be examined with an ordinary light microscope. It has been tested in several nations and confirmed to be 100% as sensitive and specific as DFA. This simple, low-cost test will be extremely useful in enhancing rabies epidemiology monitoring, particularly in underdeveloped countries where expensive fluorescence microscopes and cold storage facilities may not be accessible [22].

12.8 Lateral flow assay (immunochromatography)

The lateral flow assay is a simple and quick immunochromatographic technique. The rabies virus nucleoprotein is recognised by this test kit, which was produced utilising monoclonal antibodies. It has been tested as a quick rabies screening test.

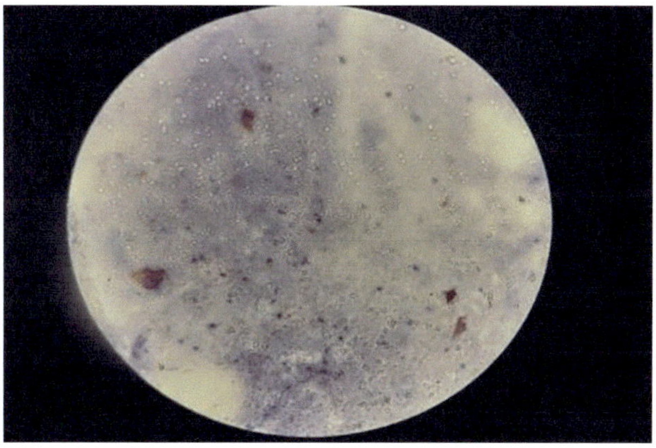

Figure 4.
Rabid animal brain impression tested by dRIT, captured by authors.

This assay is an immunodiagnostic test that provides quick findings in the field by detecting RABV antigen in post-mortem samples without the need of laboratory equipment. In summary, the detector antibodies are coupled to a membrane at two separate zones, and when the processed material is added to the device at the appropriate slot, coloured lines appear, indicating the presence of viral antigen [25].

In the case of rabies-virus-positive brain samples, coloured lines may be observed in both the 'C' (Control) and 'T' (test) zones; however, in the case of negative samples, only the 'C' zone displays colour development (**Figure 5**). Furthermore, this assay might be used to successfully identify rabies virus in cell culture [26].

12.9 Other assays for antigen detection

Other less common antigen detection techniques are as follows:

A quick sandwich ELISA is used to identify lyssaviruses belonging to all seven genotypes that circulate in Europe, Africa, Asia and Oceania [27]. Dot-blot immunoassay for brain tissues and enzyme immunoassay (EIA) for quick diagnosis in humans and animals [28].

Various PCR-based tests are now being developed for ante-mortem and post-mortem rabies diagnosis. Because the nucleoprotein (N) gene is extremely conserved, most of these PCR variants amplify it. This method has shown to be quite efficient in detecting rabies ante-mortem.

12.10 Reverse transcriptase PCR (RT-PCR)

RT-PCR tests based on gels are also used to identify rabies virus RNA in clinical samples [29–32]. The amplicons produced in these tests, notably those targeting N, G and G-L intergenic regions, have been sequenced in order to characterise the virus and analyse its phylogeny [33]. However, these assays are vulnerable to cross-contamination, which is a major problem that prevents them from being used routinely for rabies diagnosis [27].

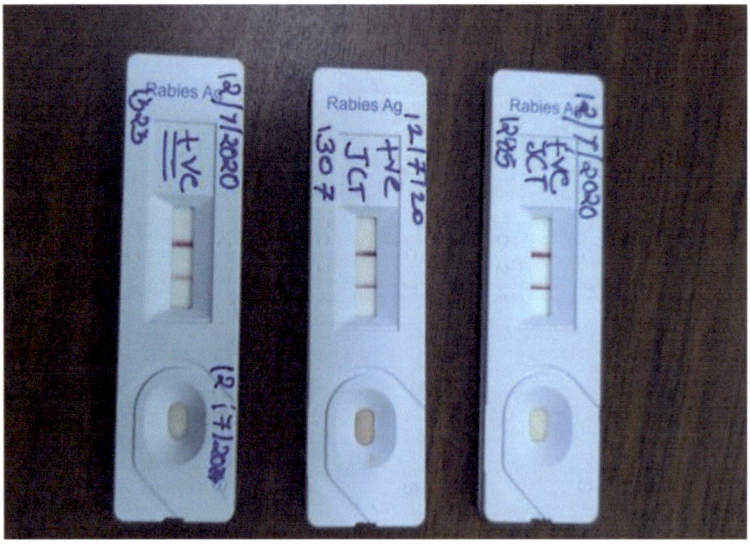

Figure 5.
Lateral flow test of rabies-positive brain sample suspensions (captured by authors).

12.11 Real-time PCR

Real-time PCR is used to identify and quantify genome copies while reducing the probability of cross-contamination. The SYBR Green real-time PCR technique is applied for rabies ante-mortem diagnosis [34] as well as finding lyssaviruses [35]. TaqMan real-time PCR tests have been shown to have high specificity [27, 36]. This was shown to be 100 times more sensitive than typical nested RT-PCR [36].

12.12 Demonstration of antibodies

Although they have certain drawbacks, the rabies virus neutralisation test, notably FAVN or RFFIT, is the test of choice for determining neutralising antibodies [37]. Various varieties of ELISA (enzyme-linked immunosorbent assay) are also utilised as an alternative since they are safe, simple and quick. Furthermore, because these tests do not involve the handling of live virus, they do not require use of high-containment facilities. The ELISA findings are shown to correspond well with the RFFIT results. ELISA based on N and G protein Mab was developed to the specially trap the rabies antigen during ante-mortem diagnosis [38].

A second-generation ELISA kit, the Platelia Rabies II, was designed to detect antibodies against the glycoprotein in blood and CSF samples. This ELISA was tested and shown to correlate well with RFFIT, making it suitable for use in laboratories without cell culture facilities [39]. However, when compared with neutralisation tests, ELISA is less sensitive [40].

13. Management of rabies

13.1 Management in human

13.1.1 Pre-exposure prophylaxis (PrEP)

PrEP (vaccination) is the most efficient way of rabies control. It not only saves the budget of the management, but it assures the prevention of the disease. There are several protocols for the prophylaxis of the disease. There are two routes for the vaccination: intra-muscular (IM) and intra-dermal (ID). Intra-dermal vaccine saves the quantity of the vaccine by 80%. The detailed protocol is given below. PrEP is recommended to the people who are associated to specific group vulnerable to rabies such as veterinarians, para-vets, animal welfare activists or people residing in endemic area. The dosage for ID is 0.1 ml at two sides while the dose of IM vaccine is whole vial. The vaccine should not be given at gluteal muscle. The protocol suggests two shots of vaccine on 0 and 7 days.

13.1.2 Post-exposure prophylaxis (PEP)

PEP is suggested after the exposure of rabies. There are three categories of the exposure listed in **Table 1**. There are three dosage regimes given by different institutions, Institut Pasteur du Cambodge regimen, Essen regimen and Zagreb regimen.

The major between immunologically naïve and previously immunised person with the PEP is no requirement of RIG in previously immunised person. The maximum dose of RIG is 20 (hRIG) or 40 (eRIG). If RIG is not available, thorough, prompt wound washing, together with immediate administration of the first vaccine dose,

Category	Immunologically naive	Previously immunised
1 Touching or feeding animals, animal licks on intact skin (no exposure)	Wash exposed skin surfaces. No PEP required.	
2 Nibbling of uncovered skin, minor scratches, or abrasions without bleeding (exposure)	Wound washing and immediate vaccination: - 2-sites ID on days 0, 3 and 7 OR - 1-site IM on days 0, 3, 7 and between days 14 and 28 OR - 2-sites IM on days 0 and 1-site IM on days 7, 21 RIG is not indicated.	Wound washing and immediate vaccination*: - 1-site ID on days 0 and 3; OR - at 4-sites ID on day 0; OR - at 1-site IM on days 0 and 3); RIG is not indicated.
3 Single or multiple transdermal bites or scratches, contamination of mucous membrane or broken skin with saliva from animal licks, exposures due to direct contact with bats (severe exposure)	Wound washing and immediate vaccination - 2-sites ID on days 0, 3 and 76 OR - 1-site IM on days 0, 3, 7 and between days 14 and 287 OR - 2-sites IM on days 0 and 1-site IM on days 7, 218 RIG administration is recommended.	Wound washing and immediate vaccination*: - 1-site ID on days 0 and 3; OR - at 4-sites ID on day 0; OR - at 1-site IM on days 0 and 3; RIG is not indicated.

Table 1.
Suggested PEP according to exposure.

followed by a complete course of rabies vaccine, is highly effective in preventing rabies. Vaccines should never be withheld, regardless of the availability of RIG. Rabies virus is enveloped virus and so through washing of bite wound with soap solution under running tap water is advised. (Adopted from [41])

13.2 Management in animals

13.2.1 Pre-exposure prophylaxis

13.2.1.1 Parenteral prophylaxis

The rabies vaccine with the potency of RIVM >2 I.U. may be used for the vaccination. The vaccine is approved for the use for the prophylaxis of apparently healthy mammals. The vaccine may be given by the IM or SC route. Generally, a temporary palpable nodule at the site of the SC injection may be noticed, which will disappear by the time. Rarely anaphylactic reaction can be seen which can be managed by SC injection of adrenalin. It is always recommended to give the vaccine a bit earlier than the due date to ensure the protection. Many a times it is possible that the whole dose of vaccine may be failed to be administered to the animals due to faulty administration. Vaccination can begin as early as 3 months of age in dogs, ferrets and livestock. Vaccines for cats can be administered as early as 2 months of age [42].

The schedule is given below in **Table 2**.

13.2.1.2 Oral prophylaxis for dogs and wildlife

The rabies vaccine bait RABORAL V-RG® contains an attenuated ('modified-live') recombinant vaccinia virus vector vaccine that expresses the rabies virus glycoprotein gene (V-RG). Since 1987, when the first licenced recombinant oral rabies vaccine (ORV) was released into the environment to immunise wildlife populations against rabies, over 250 million doses have been distributed globally with no reports of adverse responses in wildlife or domestic animals. V-RG is genetically stable, does not remain in the oral cavity for more than 48 hours after ingestion, is not shed into the environment by vaccinated animals and has been tested for thermostability in a variety of laboratory and field settings. V-RG has been tested in over 50 vertebrate species, including nonhuman primates, and no adverse effects have been reported regardless of method or dose. Immunogenicity and efficacy in a variety of target species have been established in the lab and in the field (including fox, raccoon, coyote, skunk, raccoon dog and jackal). The liquid vaccine is placed within edible baits (such as RABORAL V-RG, the vaccine-bait product) that are released into animal areas for target species to consume. The use of RABORAL V-RG in the field has helped to eradicate wildlife rabies in three European nations (Belgium, France and Luxembourg), as well as the dog/coyote rabies virus form in the United States (USA). With the final case reported in a cow in 2009, an oral rabies vaccination programme in west-central Texas has effectively removed the grey fox rabies virus strain from Texas. In the United States, a long-term ORV barrier effort using RABORAL V-RG is preventing significant geographic spread of the raccoon rabies virus strain. For more than a decade, RABORAL V-RG has been used in Israel to control wildlife rabies [44].

13.2.2 Post-exposure prophylaxis

PEP of the rabies should include five administrations of the vaccine on the days 0, 3, 7, 14, 28/90 days. If the animal is not immunised previously, eRIG is advised to be administered at the site of bite.

Species	Age at Primary Vaccination	Revaccination
Dog & Cat	After 3 months of age*	3 years**
Cattle, Horse, Sheep & Goat	After 6 months of age*	2 years**
Ferret	After 3 months of age*	1 year**

**Primary vaccination can be administered at an earlier age, but then a repeat vaccination must be given at the age of 3 or 6 months depending on the species.*
***Annual revaccination is recommended in endemic areas.*
Source: [43].

Table 2.
Vaccination schedule for animals.

14. Control of rabies

The disease is a classical example of neglected zoonosis. The disease can be well managed by the multi-disciplinary approach. Control of the rabies in the dogs is very important. World Health Organisation (WHO) has strong measures in place to prevent rabies in dogs. These guidelines include:

1. Notification of suspected cases, with euthanasia of dogs with clinical signs and those bitten by suspected rabid animals

2. Leash laws and quarantine to limit contact between susceptible dogs

3. A mass immunisation programme with ongoing boosters

4. Stray dog control and euthanasia of unvaccinated dogs roaming freely

5. Dog registration programmes [45].

Author details

Jitendrakumar Bhogilal Nayak*, Jeetendrakumar Harnathbhai Chaudhary, Prakrutik Prafulchandra Bhavsar, Pranav Ashok Anjaria, Manojbhai N. Brahmbhatt and Urvish Pravinbhai Mistry
Department of Veterinary Public Health and Epidemiology, College of Veterinary Science and Animal Husbandry, Anand Kamdhenu University, Gandhinagar, Gujarat, India

*Address all correspondence to: jbn_anand@yahoo.com

References

[1] Wilde H, Briggs DJ, Meslin FX, Hemachudha T, Sitprija V. Rabies update for travel medicine advisors. Clinical Infectious Diseases. 2003;**37**:96-100

[2] Blanton JD, Rupprecht CE. Travel vaccination for rabies. Expert Review of Vaccines. 2008;**7**:613-620

[3] Kuzmin IV, Mayer AE, Niezgoda M, Markotter W, et al. Shimoni bat virus, a new representative of the lyssavirus genus. Virus Research. 2010;**149**:197-210

[4] Bourhy H, Dautry-Varsat A, Hotez PJ, Salomon J. Rabies, still neglected after 125 years of vaccination. PLoS Neglected Tropical Diseases. 2010;**4**:e839

[5] Knobel DL, Cleaveland S, Coleman PG, Fèvre EM, et al. Re-evaluating the burden of rabies in Africa and Asia. Bulletin of the World Health Organization. 2005;**83**:360-368

[6] Baer GM. The history of rabies. In: Rabies. London: Academic Press; 2007. pp. 1-22

[7] Giesen A, Gniel D, Malerczyk C. 30 years of rabies vaccination with Rabipur: A summary of clinical data and global experience. Expert Review of Vaccines. 2015;**14**:351-367

[8] Bernard H-U, Burk RD, Chen Z, Van Doorslaer K, Al E. Classification of papillomaviruses (PVs) based on 189 PV types and proposal of taxonomic amendments. Virology. 2012;**401**:70-79

[9] Constable PD, Done SH, and Walter Grunberg KWH. VETERINARY: A Textbook of the Diseases of Cattle, Horses, Sheep, Pigs, and Goats VetBooks. Diseases of the Nervous System. Peter DC, Kenneth W, Hinchcliff, Stanley HD, Walter Grünberg, editors. 11th edition. Veterinary Medicine. W.B. Saunders; 2017:1155-1370. DOI: 10.1016/B978-0-7020-5246-0.00014-0. Available from: https://www.sciencedirect.com/science/article/pii/B9780702052460000140. ISBN: 9780702052460.

[10] Rupprecht CE. Rhabdoviruses: Rabies Virus. USA: University of Texas, Medical Branch at Galveston; 1996

[11] Kuzmin IV. An arctic fox rabies virus strain as the cause of human rabies in Russian Siberia. Archives of Virology. 1999;**144**:627-629

[12] Singh R, Singh KP, Cherian S, Saminathan M, et al. Rabies – Epidemiology, pathogenesis, public health concerns and advances in diagnosis and control: A comprehensive review. The Veterinary Quarterly. 2017;**37**:212-251

[13] Yousaf MZ, Qasim M, Zia S, Rehman Khan M, et al. Rabies molecular virology, diagnosis, prevention and treatment. Virology Journal. 2012;**9**(1):1-5. Available from: https://virologyj.biomedcentral.com/articles/10.1186/1743-422X-9-50

[14] Chhabra M, Ichhpujani RL, Tewari KN, Lal S. Human Rabies in Delhi. Indian Journal of Pediatrics. 2004;**71**:217-220

[15] Tharp TA. Rabies: Assessing Rabies Spread Determinants. Doctoral dissertation. San Diego: University of California; 2016

[16] Salomão C, Nacima A, Cuamba L, Gujral L, et al. Epidemiology, clinical features and risk factors for human rabies and animal bites during an outbreak of rabies in Maputo and Matola cities,

Mozambique, 2014: Implications for public health interventions for rabies control. PLoS Neglected Tropical Diseases. 2017;**11**(7):1-16

[17] Global elimination of dog-mediated human rabies - The Time Is Now! - OIE - World Organisation for Animal Health n.d.

[18] Coleman PG, Dye C. Immunization coverage required to prevent outbreaks of dog rabies. Vaccine. 1996;**14**:185-186

[19] Centers for Disease Control and Prevention, How is rabies transmitted? | Transmission | CDC 2019

[20] Ngoepe CE, Sabeta C, Nel L. The spread of canine rabies into Free State province of South Africa: A molecular epidemiological characterization. Virus Research. 2009;**142**:175-180

[21] Khalafalla AI, Ali YH. Rabies virus infection in livestock. In: Rabies virus at the beginning of 21st century. IntechOpen; 2021. DOI: 10.5772/intechopen.98228

[22] Isloor S, Sharada R, Rahaman SA. Rabies. In RK, Malik Yashpal Singh D.K, Singh, editors. Animal-Origin Viral Zoonoses. Singapore: Springer; DOI: 10.1007/978-981-15-2651-0_1

[23] Meslin FX, Kaplan MM, Koprowski H. World Health Organization. Laboratory techniques in rabies. World Health Organization. 1973. Available from: https://apps.who.int/iris/handle/10665/38286

[24] Stear MJ. OIE manual of diagnostic tests and vaccines for terrestrial animals. Parasitology. 2005;**130**:727-727

[25] Kang BK, Oh JS, Lee CS, Park BK, et al. Evaluation of a rapid immunodiagnostic test kit for rabies virus. Journal of Virological Methods. 2007;**145**:30-36

[26] Sharada R, Veeresh BH, Palaniappan C, Sekhar B, et al. A novel approach through application of lateral flow assay (immunochromatography) for detection of rabies virus in the cell culture harvest.Commonwealth Veterinary Journal. 2015;**31**(2):5-8

[27] Mani RS, Madhusudana SN. Laboratory diagnosis of human rabies: Recent advances. Scientific World Journal. 2013;**2013**. Available from: https://www.hindawi.com/journals/tswj/2013/569712. DOI: 10.1155/2013/569712

[28] Vasanth JP, Madhusudana SN, Abhilash KV, Suja MS, Muhamuda K. Development and evaluation of an enzyme immunoassay for rapid diagnosis of rabies in humans and animals. Indian Journal of Pathology & Microbiology. 2004;**47**:574-578

[29] Ratho RK, Biswal M, Mishra B. Role of reverse transcriptase polymerase chain reaction for the diagnosis of human rabies. The Indian Journal of Medical Research. 2012;**135**:837-842

[30] Crepin P, Audry L, Rotivel Y, Gacoin A, et al. Intravitam diagnosis of human rabies by PCR using saliva and cerebrospinal fluid. Journal of Clinical Microbiology. 1998;**36**:1117-1121

[31] Dacheux L, Reynes JM, Buchy P, Sivuth O, et al. A reliable diagnosis of human rabies based on analysis of skin biopsy specimens. Clinical Infectious Diseases. 2008;**47**:1410-1417

[32] Coertse J, Weyer J, Nel LH, Markotter W. Improved PCR methods for detection of african rabies and rabies-related lyssaviruses. Journal of Clinical Microbiology. 2010;**48**:3949-3955

[33] Pramina K, Veeresh B, Isloor SI, Rathnamma D, et al. Genetic variability

of the G-L intergenic region sequences of Indian rabies virus strains circulating in animals. International Journal of Infectious Diseases. 2016;**45**:238

[34] Nagaraj T, Vasanth JP, Desai A, Kamat A, et al. Ante mortem diagnosis of human rabies using saliva samples: Comparison of real time and conventional RT-PCR techniques. Journal of Clinical Virology. 2006;**36**:17-23

[35] Hayman DTS, Banyard AC, Wakeley PR, Harkess G, et al. A universal real-time assay for the detection of lyssaviruses. Journal of Virological Methods. 2011;**177**:87-93

[36] Wakeley PR, Johnson N, McElhinney LM, Marston D, et al. Development of a real-time, TaqMan reverse transcription-PCR assay for detection and differentiation of lyssavirus genotypes 1, 5, and 6. Journal of Clinical Microbiology. 2005;**43**:2786-2792

[37] Sunilkumar KM, Isloor S, Kamran CA, Santosh AK, et al. Sero monitoring of anti rabies vaccinal antibodies to pep in animals by RFFIT - a case study in Karnataka. Journal of Experimental Biology and Agricultural Sciences. 2016;**4**:S103-S107

[38] Muhamuda K, Madhusudana SN, Ravi V. Development and evaluation of a competitive ELISA for estimation of rabies neutralizing antibodies after post-exposure rabies vaccination in humans. International Journal of Infectious Diseases. 2007;**11**:441-445

[39] Feyssaguet M, Dacheux L, Audry L, Compoint A, et al. Multicenter comparative study of a new ELISA, PLATELIA™ RABIES II, for the detection and titration of anti-rabies glycoprotein antibodies and comparison with the rapid fluorescent focus inhibition test (RFFIT) on human samples from vaccinated and non-vacc. Vaccine. 2007;**25**:2244-2251

[40] Cliquet F, McElhinney LM, Servat A, Boucher JM, et al. Development of a qualitative indirect ELISA for the measurement of rabies virus-specific antibodies from vaccinated dogs and cats. Journal of Virological Methods. 2004;**117**:1-8

[41] World Health Organization. Rabies vaccines: WHO position paper, April 2018 – Recommendations. Vaccine. 2018;**36**:5500-5503

[42] CDC—Veterinarians: Rabies Vaccination—Rabies. n.d

[43] Nobivac® Rabies—MSD Animal Health India. n.d

[44] Maki J, Guiot AL, Aubert M, Brochier B, et al. Oral vaccination of wildlife using a vaccinia-rabies-glycoprotein recombinant virus vaccine (RABORAL V-RG®): A global review. Veterinary Research. 2017;**48**:1-26

[45] Rupprecht CE. Rabies in Dogs. 2018. Available from: https://www.msdvetmanual.com/dog-owners/brain,-spinal-cord,-and-nerve-disorders-of-dogs/rabies-in-dogs

Chapter 4

Implications of COVID-19 on Public Policy, Supply Chain Disruptions, and Monitoring Methods

Timothy J. Tse, Farley Chicilo, Jeffrey Popiel and Martin J.T. Reaney

Abstract

Transmission of the severe acute respiratory syndrome coronavirus 2, referred to as COVID-19, has persisted beyond 2020 and led to a global pandemic with far reaching consequences. Many changes in public policy and health measures were developed and implemented with the intention of slowing the spread of the novel virus. Disruptions from the global pandemic created major supply chain consequences due to stockpiling of essential goods (alcohol-based hand sanitizers and surface disinfectants), impacts on trade routes, and limitations on modes of transportation due to border closures. Rapid increase in the use of hand sanitizers and surface disinfectants significantly affected the production capacity of high-quality ethanol (e.g., USP and FCC grade) resulting in regulatory changes in countries facing shortages. Prompt enactment of government policies allowed for use of alcohol with higher impurities to offset heightened demand and increase commercial availability. Changes in monitoring methods were also observed, where many agencies began to track viral shedding through municipal wastewater. In this chapter, we will discuss the impacts of COVID-19 on public policies and health measures, economics as it relates to supply chain disruptions, and the implementation of novel monitoring methods to survey the spread of COVID-19.

Keywords: COVID-19, public policy, monitoring methods, hand sanitizer, surface disinfectant, pandemic

1. Introduction

The emergence of severe acute respiratory syndrome coronavirus 2 (SARS-CoV-2; aka. COVID-19) has led to unprecedented global responses in the attempt to limit and slow propagation of the virus. These responses included the shutdown of major manufacturing plants [1], limitations on social gatherings, travel and transportation restrictions, enacting state of emergencies, and public health measures (e.g., social distancing, use of face coverings and hygienic practices, closures of non-essential businesses and schools, and vaccine mandates) [2]. Even with the development and implementation of safe and effective vaccines, and continued efforts to prevent transmission among the public, COVID-19 has persisted in spreading globally, and new more virulent variants have evolved.

The enactment of public policy restrictions, including social distancing, travel restrictions, access to testing, and contact tracing initiatives decreased COVID-19 infection, morbidity, and mortality rates [3, 4]. Such policies and tools were especially effective in slowing transmission and reducing the strain on healthcare facilities that have been stretched beyond their typical operating capacity [5]. Many governments implemented a variety of technologies, incentives, and practices to track infection, promote vaccination, and enforce restrictions [6]. Biomolecular approaches (e.g., nucleic acid amplification tests) were also implemented to help provide quantitative numbers to investigate spread and infection rates. Altogether, these technologies were implemented to slow the spread of infection and provide strategic advice for informing public health policies.

Unfortunately, economic recovery from the COVID-19 pandemic has been slow, primarily due to supply chain disruptions that have led to low inventories, employment layoffs, and reductions in industrial production and services [1]. Furthermore, as restrictions began to ease, formerly constrained demand for consumer goods surged beyond manufacturing capacity. With diminished inventory and a weakened shipping industry, recovery was slow, and meeting consumer demand became challenging [7]. The demand for antiseptics and medical supplies increased significantly while supply chain constraints intensified. Faced with shortages governments and municipalities implemented impromptu solutions for increasing regional production of much needed hand sanitizers [8]. One effective response was the introduction of legislation that allowed the use of lower-grades of ethanol (often technical-grade ethanol) in the formulation of disinfectant and sanitizing products [8–10].

As the COVID-19 pandemic waned and vaccination limited the severity of viral infection, many governments removed restrictions and opted for more permissive policies that allowed citizens to live with a higher risk of contracting the virus. Health policies designed to reduce transmission among the public were mitigated or ceased altogether. With the implementation of gradual re-opening measures in many countries, policies defining travel restrictions, social distancing, facial coverings, etc. were removed through the 2nd, 3rd, and 4th quarters of 2021, and first quarter of 2022 [2]. Direct monitoring methods for COVID-19 (e.g., contact tracing and biomolecular tests) were also removed during the relaxation of restrictions. For example, Germany ceased free covid testing in August of 2021 with the acknowledgement that testing was both expensive and specifically benefitted the unvaccinated [11]. Currently, many monitoring methods have now targeted wastewater-based epidemiology (WBE) studies to survey the spread of infection in different communities [12–18]. Although these methods can provide early detection [19–22], interpretation of data can be limited in scope when compared with testing of populations, as is discussed below.

Finally, with continued policy changes, the economic recovery due to the COVID-19 pandemic has been slow. GDP dropped sharply across the globe at the start of the pandemic but rebounded somewhat shortly after. Global GDP at the end of 2020 was only a few percentage points less year-over-year than at the end of 2021 [23]. Worldwide merchandise trade decreased significantly, while trade of medical goods increased. Nearly all industries managed to recover by the end of 2021, with transportation & warehousing, tourism, and live entertainment-based industries

DOI: http://dx.doi.org/10.5772/intechopen.105805

having yet to return to pre-pandemic levels [24, 25]. Late pandemic supply chain disruptions have shown that pre-pandemic conditions have not returned [26, 27]. With continued risk of future supply-chain catastrophes, some in business are moving to models that develop localized value chains. The purpose of this book chapter is to discuss and review the impacts of COVID-19 on public policy, health measures, economic disruptions, and the importance of surveillance methods for the early detection of infections.

2. Economic disruptions and supply chain shortages, including ethanol-based products

The economic contraction that occurred during the COVID-19 pandemic affected global markets in 2020, 2021, and into 2022. Prominent among economic challenges were supply chain disruptions, which broadly impacted the delivery of goods and services. For example, manufacturers, builders, and retailers had reduced or delayed access to input materials, building materials, and stock items [9, 26]. Sales sharply decreased as pandemic-related restrictions were introduced in March 2020 which led to an excess of inventory. In some cases, this inventory was written off or liquidated. In later stages of the pandemic in 2021–2022, economic recovery placed additional stress on markets. Manufacturing industries halted or reduced output, canceled orders, and reduced reorders which led to manufacturing that was retooled or refocused to provide goods that were in high demand [26].

Among supply shortages, much of the world's consumers and businesses had challenges acquiring antiseptics such as rubbing alcohol, hand sanitizer, antiseptic wipes, and surface disinfectants at the beginning of the pandemic, which was exacerbated by consumer hoarding [9]. Due to the circumstances of limited world-wide supply of United States Pharmacopeia (USP) or Food-Chemicals Codex (FCC) grade ethanol, Canada modified acceptance criteria to include ethanol that was produced by alternative methods with specific label and usage requirements [28]. Health Canada expedited processing of Site Licenses and Product Licenses for hand sanitizer manufacturing and sales and waived the need for a review of good manufacturing practices (GMP) for new manufacturers, requiring only a signed declaration instead of the usual full GMP documentation [29]. Hand sanitizer supply expanded quickly with the new regulations, and shortages were rapidly addressed. Unfortunately, many producers failed to meet quality standards for ethanol as defined by new regulations [9]. In addition to supporting production of hand sanitizer, Health Canada expedited applications for Drug Identification Numbers (DIN) allowing the sale of surface disinfectants [30].

Worldwide lockdowns contributed to production and acquisition challenges by exacerbating industry down-time and supply-chain shortages, leading to cascading delays [26]. For many businesses the early response to Covid was a strategic long-term decrease in production achieved by layoffs, and a reduction of parts and other inputs (e.g., semiconductors for automakers) [26]. The shipping industry followed this pattern by reducing schedules.

After lockdown restrictions began to ease there was an unanticipated surge of product orders, combined with reduced capacity, making responding to new demand difficult [1]. Many laid off workers decided not to return to their positions through resignation, and retirement. These social factors lead to a labour shortage [31, 32]. In Canada the unemployment rate increased to 9.5%. This represents the loss of almost one million jobs in 2021 [23]. In the United States of America (U.S.A.) record numbers of resignations occurred in 2021, with 4.4 million workers resigning [33]. Employee resignations occurred for multiple reasons: while some workers planned to avoid potential workplace COVID-19 infection (Delta and Omicron variants), others were faced with lifestyle choices related to the epidemic and other pandemic-related stresses, such as reduced availability of childcare and elder care services [33]. Indeed, a large cohort of "baby boomers" simply chose to retire. Continuing resignations required extra resources used in hiring, onboarding and offboarding, thereby decreasing the efficiency of businesses and further contributing to industrial disruptions [33]. The job market became increasingly competitive with a new human resource focus on retention strategies [33].

Any business with a complex supply chain was susceptible to production backlogs, which resulted in backorders of inputs and delayed product shipments [23]. Freight costs more than doubled by the end of 2020, with smaller businesses being impacted more significantly, receiving lower priorities due to lower volume orders and higher shipping rates than larger companies with long-term contracts [34]. Tourism-based industries, such as hotels, restaurants, the arts and entertainment, recreation, and travel, diminished quickly when stay-at-home measures were put in place to limit COVID-19 transmission [23]. Once public health measures were lifted, there was a record number of job openings in 2021 due to the quick rise in job availability from impacted industries returning to regular business operations [23]. Through 2021, tourism-based industries exhibited the slowest recovery since the beginning of the pandemic, with transportation and warehousing as the next slowest, showing 16% below pre-pandemic GDP levels in Canada from February 2020 to January 2022, whereas most other industries achieved full GDP recovery [24].

To add to the economic challenges caused by the pandemic, the state of Texas had temperatures dip below freezing with snowfall in late February 2021 [35]. Chemical and petrochemical supply chains were heavily affected, as Texas is the nation's leading producer, and this extraordinary weather system caused major disruptions across the state [35]. Manufacturing facilities in these industries took months to recover [35] and as a result, industries involving plastics, packaging, fertilizers, pesticides, synthetic fibers, cleaners, lubricants, paint, and many more were affected by reduced supply in a market that was already suffering from supply backlogs [35].

In the U.S.A., high demand for import shipments quickly created a shortage of drayage vehicles and drivers while freight value moved by all transport vehicles fell 9.1 percent year over year from 2019 to 2020 [26, 34]. Although this year-over-year decrease is significant, it does not show the extreme swing of GDP in the first three quarters of 2020 as compared between **Figures 1** and **2**. Exports from Canada to the U.S.A. decreased by 70 billion dollars (16%) and imports by 43 billion dollars (11%) [23]. By the end of 2020 the U.S.A. and Canadian economies saw an overall contraction, despite significant recovery in the third quarter, owing to significantly decreased trade between U.S.A. and Canada [23, 25].

Worldwide merchandise trade decreased by 7% in 2020 [38], while the trade of medical goods increased, as demand for PPE (personal protective equipment) and other medical items (ventilators, AEDs, various consumables, drugs) escalated [39]. The first lockdown (and economic contraction) started in China, with lockdowns occurring months before those enacted elsewhere in the world [2]. This afforded China the ability to experience an economic expansion in the 2nd quarter of 2020, as seen in **Figure 2**.

DOI: http://dx.doi.org/10.5772/intechopen.105805

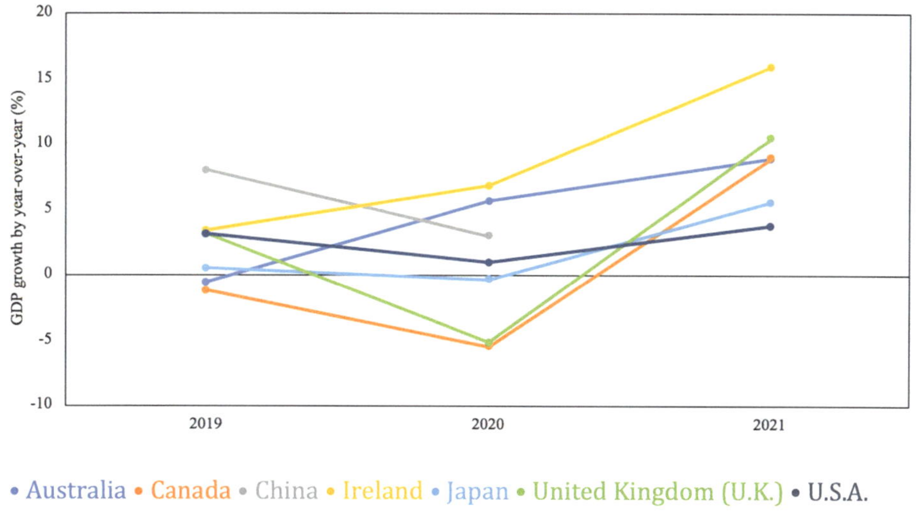

Figure 1.
GDP growth expressed in % change year-over-year. Reconstructed from [36].

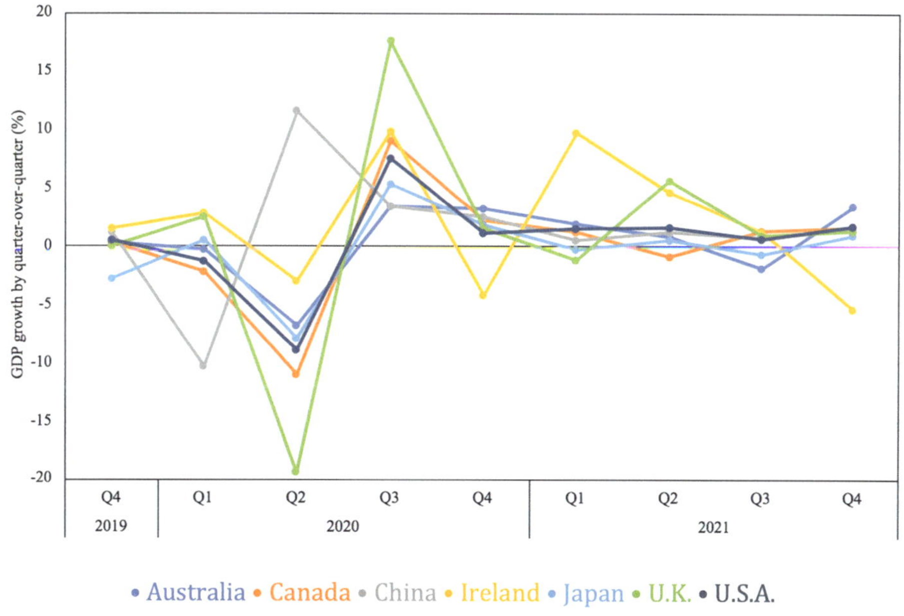

Figure 2.
GDP growth expressed in % change quarter-over-quarter. Reconstructed from [37].

Despite the short-term risks of using a lean, or 'just-in-time' approach to doing business, economists see value in maintaining its use [40]. It is possible that the economy may have maintained stability for a longer period if it had used more supply reserves, but the supply required to outlast the continued demand would have been insurmountable in many cases, as any physical product requires a reliable influx of materials to match output; a larger stock merely acts as a longer-lasting buffer to ease supply shock.

Economists have been analyzing and formulating potential solutions to avoid economic contractions like those experienced in 2020 [41]. It has been speculated that putting less reliance on international supply chains and focusing on more local value chains might increase economic loss and create more vulnerabilities in domestic economies [39]. Each country has their own specialized industries and products and continued association to these markets allows for optimal economic gains. In contrast, this interconnectivity also increases the potential negative impacts resulting from global supply chain issues, suggesting a need for more economic self-sufficiency [27]. Relying on a globalized economy may show some benefit, but only in the long-term, and such reliance leaves industries in a vulnerable position in the case of worldwide or specific supplier-affecting disruptions, especially for businesses with complex supply chains.

3. Public healthcare policies

The onset of the COVID-19 pandemic in early 2020 forced governments across the globe to act quickly to reshape public health policy. A major effort to alleviate the stress on health care was described as a "flatten the curve" strategy, but ultimately this approach recognized that the spread of the virus could be slowed but not stopped [42]. Indeed, the spread of the virus continued throughout 2021, and into 2022. In response, governments, health care agencies, and private industries have continued to enact public health measures to mitigate the spread of the virus and its effects. Public health measures have included mandating behavioral practices (social distancing, limited gathering sizes, etc.) [43], use of hygienic products (hand sanitizers, masking) [9], travel restrictions [44], and modifications to the delivery of health care services (online doctors' visits, postponement of elective surgery) [45]. Rates of COVID-associated morbidity and mortality are proportional to the amount of circulating COVID-19 virus within a population, and as of May 2022, total COVID-19 associated deaths are estimated to be more than 6.27 million [46]. This staggering loss of human life highlights the necessity of effective public health policy to minimize infection. Multiple peaks of global COVID-19 deaths were observed from 2022 to 2022. Such waves were often preceded by lower case numbers which, in turn, can cause complacency among the public. However, the emergence of increasingly

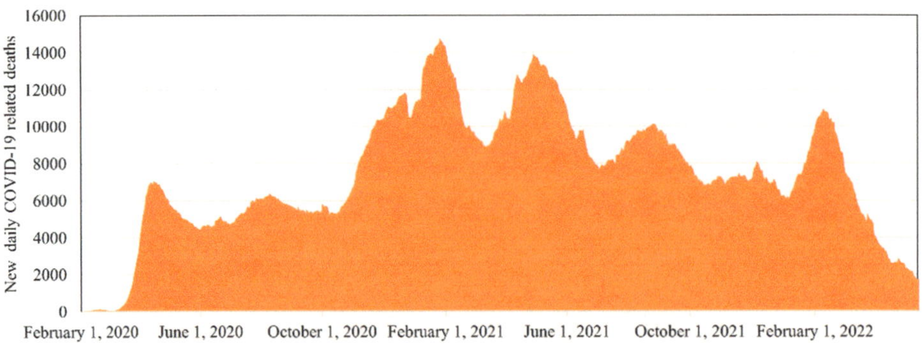

Figure 3.
Global figures of new deaths from February 1, 2020, to may 15, 2022. New COVID-19 deaths reported show patterns of repeated waves of outbreaks across the world as the pandemic progressed. Reconstructed from [46].

contagious strains of COVID-19, such as the Delta and Omicron variants, make the pandemic likely to continue into the foreseeable future (**Figure 3**).

The COVID-19 pandemic has had devastating and lasting effects on the health care system. The resulting increase in hospitalization rates and diminished resources available to treat patients has added significant burden to an already strained system. Policies designed to increase available ventilators [47], intensive care unit (ICU) beds [48], access to COVID-19 testing kits, and vaccination have been important tools that governments have enacted to fight the ongoing pandemic and minimize loss of life. Unfortunately, policies cannot address the immediate need for additional health care workers as it takes many years of training and specialization to care for patients, especially those in critical care settings [49].

To combat avoidable and unnecessary hospitalizations, well-enforced behavioral policies, such as social distancing and face masks, are often quickly enacted, as they do not overly disrupt economic and social systems and have demonstrated effectiveness in reducing transmission [50]. Reducing viral transmission via face-to-face interactions leads to an overall decrease in hospitalization rates. Most critically, this reduction extends to those who are at the highest risk for COVID-associated morbidity and mortality, such as individuals with underlying health care issues and patients over the age of 65 [51]. Public policy involving social distancing has taken various forms, ranging from severe restrictions on personal movement, to limited or no restrictions at all. Importantly, travel restrictions and encouragement of virtual or teleworking, helps limit travel and public contact, something that many in the workforce were able to do effectively during the COVID-19 pandemic [51–53]. Teleworking practices have the added benefit of reducing non-essential travel both internationally and domestically, which delays transmission of the virus. Indeed, there is strong evidence that restrictions on international travel from countries with high infection rates helps in slowing the spread of COVID-19 [44]. To eliminate avoidable public transmission, China imposed drastic lockdowns as outbreaks emerged throughout the country, including restricting travel from other nations, and between regions [54]. Chinese restrictions extended to include the separation of family members in the case of diagnosed infections. India suffered devastating infection rates during April and May of 2021 and imposed district specific restrictions during the second wave of infections to help mitigate the spread through densely populated regions [55]. In the United States and Canada, restrictions and guidelines varied significantly from region to region, owing to local policies, population density, and infection rates. Evidence in the United States suggests that stricter enforcement of public policy measures is likely linked to lower infection rates [56], while sudden, removal of restrictions has led to additional outbreaks [55, 57, 58]. Many governments chose to enact "phases" of restrictions, which lead to gradual policy changes intended to ease the stress on both public and private health care systems by controlling the total number of cases.

Hygienic methods such as hand washing, use of sanitizers, and implementation of personal protective equipment (PPE) have also been shown to be effective at reducing transmission of the COVID-19 virus. Although hand washing is a highly effective practice, the use of hand sanitizers was found to be substantially more convenient than hand washing. The resulting high demand for alcohol-based sanitizers, as well as other essential supplies, led to global shortages [9, 59]. The consequences of these shortages are still being studied, but food and supply scarcities are likely to cause an increase in prices, which disproportionately affect those with lower socioeconomic status [60]. To try and combat shortages, governments have encouraged sourcing from local suppliers while trying to minimize disruptions to essential imports.

Even so, supply chain issues can be particularly challenging in rural populations where food security is already an issue [61].

Large, population-scale testing was implemented as a major intervention strategy to manage COVID-19 infections across the world as community infections increased. Improved access to testing allows for earlier identification of infections, encouraging individuals to self-quarantine and slow the spread of COVID-19. However, difficulties in acquiring testing methods, and significant delays in obtaining results, were frequent criticisms of large-scale testing efforts [62]. If wait times for testing are exceedingly long, individuals are less likely to test. Likewise, the longer the wait between preforming a test and obtaining the results, the less likely an individual will isolate, particularly if they are asymptomatic [63]. Mass testing can be costly, and so testing of health-care workers, symptomatic individuals, and those who are at risk of serious health complications are prioritized. Further exacerbating testing issues was a shortage of reagents, which caused supply chain issues and contributed to the wide disparities of testing rates between countries [64, 65]. A proposed solution to reduce the use of testing supplies is the pooling of samples, allowing for multiple individuals to be tested simultaneously by combining samples and testing with a single reaction. If the result from the pooled samples is negative, then all subsequent individuals are considered negative. However, if a positive result is observed, then individuals are tested separately, reducing the strain on the testing process. Remarkably, Chinese authorities in the city of Qingdao were able to test over seven million people over the course of three days using the method of pooling samples [66]. While the pooling method has demonstrated efficiency, there are limitations to the technique, including the need for relatively low positivity rates, longer reporting delays [63], and a reduction in test sensitivity [67]. Another frequently used method to determine community positivity rates is the testing of wastewater, which can predict general infection rates and is discussed in greater detail below.

Restrictions stemming from public policies can have far reaching impacts, and so constraints and policy changes must be carefully considered to prevent unnecessary disruptions to the economy, crucial supply chains, and earnings by those who are disproportionately affected by the pandemic [68]. Throughout the COVID-19 pandemic, health care experts have advocated for the enactment and enforcement of public health policies, imposing restrictions on social distancing, face coverings in public settings (especially where social distancing may not be possible), respiratory hygiene, and, where necessary, lockdowns [69]. There is evidence that demographic factors such as race, gender, and socioeconomic conditions play a role in transmission, contraction, and overall mortality rates and so not all measures are equally effective [51, 70, 71]. Critically, stay at home orders have adverse effects on supply chain issues, employment, and mental health [72, 73]. Research has shown that the practice of social distancing has caused negative impacts on isolation [74], family stresses [75], domestic violence [76], consumption of alcohol [77], and mental health [78], and so preventative and behavioral policies should be considered before major shutdowns of schools, businesses, and strict stay at home orders are enforced. Many factors play a role in COVID-19 related infections, and government policies should be careful to consider the effectiveness, financial costs, and negative outcomes associated with the policy enforcement. The development and distribution of safe and effective vaccines has helped to reduce the number of deaths and the pressures on hospital systems [79], however higher vaccination rates are concentrated in higher income countries, and vaccination hesitancy, along with the emergence of new more virulent COVID-19 variants, can slow development of broad spread immunity [80]. The consequence of the continued spread of the virus indicates that the COVID-19 pandemic is likely far from over, and public policies will serve as an effective tool in reducing transmission in the future.

4. Infection tracking and surveillance

A variety of technologies have emerged to alleviate the temporal and social restrictions brought on by the COVID-19 pandemic. These include the use of artificial intelligence (medical tracking), social media platforms (creating awareness of infections and providing real-time updates), virtual and augmented reality communications, blockchain (integration of point-of-care diagnostics for self-testing), additive manufacturing (production of personal protective equipment), 5G cellular technology and smart applications (remote monitoring of COVID-19), geographical information systems (spatial tracking of COVID-19), and autonomous robots (use of drones for disinfection) [6]. These valuable technologies provided critical information regarding COVID-19 and offered alternative communication means for health-related and employment-related meetings.

To manage the spread of COVID-19, other unprecedented techniques were adopted including contact tracing and the use of digital technologies [3, 4] as well as initiatives to provide early detection, monitoring efforts, and surveillance technologies. These technologies were introduced to slow and contain the spread of COVID-19 and provide advisory bodies important details in making informed public health strategies to combat the virus.

Contact tracing involves the identification of individuals who have come into close contact with an infected person, testing them, and, in case of an infection, tracing their own contacts to reduce the spread of an infection throughout a population [81]. Unfortunately, traditional manual contact tracing is labor-intensive, time-consuming, and may not be adequate in monitoring for COVID-19 in real time, especially in the instance of high infection rates [82]. Consequently, the development of digital tracking apps, including contact tracing apps (CTAs), have garnered attention in early detection by combining proximity tracing and contact tracing [3]. These novels CTAs, such as Canada's COVID Alert app [83], rely on self-reporting from infected individuals, as well as the implementation of Bluetooth connectivity to measure and record the spatial proximity between users, and alert nearby persons if they are within proximity to an infected individual [3]. Unfortunately, these applications are technologically limited as they can raise privacy concerns and older smartphones may not be compatible. Digital applications such as CTAs can also exacerbate inequities, such as age and income discrepancies in accessing smartphones, which can ultimately lead to a decline in CTAs effectiveness in preventing the spread of COVID-19 [3]. Another unforeseen occurrence resulting from the use of CTAs comes from a significant increase in the volume of people who receive notifications after being in close proximity of a COVID-19 positive individual. A dramatic surge of notifications was observed by contact tracing apps in the UK in July 2021, where the total number of individuals notified increased by nearly 50% in a single week. This surge in CTA alerts resulted in what was coined the "pingdemic" and required those affected to self-isolate for 10 days [84]. This caused significant consequences for many industries, including manufacturing and hospitality, as hundreds of thousands of individuals were required to stay home, leading to the shutdown of several production lines [84].

With the gradual lifting of social and travel restrictions, and the reopening of borders, access to PCR testing for COVID-19 has subsided and measuring an accurate clinical picture of the spread of the virus has become increasingly more difficult [85]. This has, however, paved the way for wastewater testing to play an increasingly critical role in monitoring for COVID-19 transmission within communities [85]. Currently, there are 5 genes that have routinely been used to screen for the presence of COVID-19. These include the ORF1ab, E-, N-, S-, and the RNA dependent RNA polymerase (RdRp) genes [86–88], encoding for numerous structural and non-structural proteins. Specifically, the RdRp gene is essential for the replication and transcription of the virus, and is encoded by the open reading frame, ORF1ab gene. In addition, ORF1ab is the largest gene that encodes for several nonstructural proteins [89]. Meanwhile, The E-, N-, and S- genes encode for structural proteins including, envelope proteins, nucleocapsid proteins, and spike proteins, respectively [90–92].

Recently, WBE studies have been employed to monitor the spread of COVID-19. Wastewater infrastructure is an important component of early warning systems to detect disease, due to increased water usage for hygienic purposes (hand washing, disinfection, cleaning, etc.) [19]. As COVID-19 and viral RNA are shed in bodily excreta (saliva, feces, sputum) of infected individuals [93], detection in wastewater [94] can provide early warnings and infer trends for authorities to make informed decisions on public policies and restrictions [19–22].

WBE studies [16, 17] have been used in several countries including Italy, Netherlands, Portugal, Spain, Australia, China, France, Israel, United States, Turkey, and Canada [12–15]. These studies typically involve the extraction of viral RNA material and amplifying the nucleic acid to detect the presence of COVID-19 (i.e., Nucleic acid amplification tests; NAATs, quantitative polymerase chain reaction; qPCR, reverse transcriptase PCR; RT-PCR, etc.) [95], and are important in evaluating the spread, genetic diversity, and geographic distribution of the virus [94, 96]. WBE modeling can be used to provide an estimate on the number of infected individuals in a population based on: (1) concentration of COVID-19 RNA at the inlet of the wastewater treatment plant, (2) volumetric flow rate of the wastewater treatment plant, (3) fecal load, (4) RNA shedding in the stool, and (5) RNA losses in the sewer pipe [97]. For the sensitive detection of viruses in wastewater, samples are often concentrated before quantification [98, 99]. For the surveillance of COVID-19, wastewater samples are often concentrated using centrifugation [100], filtration [101–105], polyethylene glycol precipitation [103, 106, 107], or aluminum flocculation [108, 109]. Unfortunately, RNA extraction efficiency can vary due to co-concentration of organic compounds (e.g., humic substances) [12]. Recent studies of COVID-19 in wastewater have also observed viral recoveries between 3 and 50% [12], although calibration against RNA losses in the wastewater can provide improved accuracy [97]. Nonetheless, these techniques have demonstrated reliability in identifying the true magnitude of infection within a population [97] and have been widely used to monitor for early detection of novel viral pathogens [110–113], including enterovirus, adenoviruses, hepatitis viruses, and more recently COVID-19. As WBE assesses changes in SAR-CoV-2 titres, these studies collectively include asymptomatic individuals, as well as those exhibiting very mild symptoms. Unfortunately, translation of COVID-19 titres in wastewater to actual individual numbers is extremely difficult. Therefore, these analyses are typically used to infer the spread of COVID-19 within a community and monitor for the emergence of related variants.

While PCR tests performed on wastewater samples are identical to those performed at COVID-19 clinics, the N- and E-genes are more commonly targeted as they are more well-preserved in wastewater [85]. However, there are challenges with wastewater testing, including variability of the data produced by each sample which can produce a significant margin of error [85]. Furthermore, the operations and designs among different wastewater treatment facilities can result in varying dilutions of the tested samples, thus affecting signals of COVID-19 in the wastewater [114, 115]. For example, in some facilities, rainfall may combine with wastewater, resulting in the dilution of COVID-19. Additionally, residential, and industrial water uses can affect COVID-19 signals in municipal wastewater. Therefore, comparing COVID-19 levels between different communities, cities, health regions, etc. is very difficult and wastewater analyses for COVID-19 should be primarily used to establish trends in COVID-19 prevalence, rather than determining an absolute concentration or comparing to active cases in the community; active cases may not include asymptomatic individuals, whereas wastewater analyses will.

Altogether, wastewater surveillance of COVID-19 provides a powerful tool in evaluating incidences of disease at the community level. However, WBE studies also need to be integrated into other public health studies, such as randomized testing of individuals. Current data on COVID-19 and other viruses suggest that WBE epidemiology is a viable option in assessing and mitigating viral outbreaks [12–17]. The widely used q(RT)-PCR approach enables rapid and strain level RNA/DNA quantification, however, the primers and probes should be chosen carefully, depending on sequence preservation [90–92]. Finally, targeted, and untargeted sequencing of viruses in wastewater has the potential to track the spread of specific sequence variants and identify mutations that could affect detection in clinical settings [12] and provide early detection for emergence of novel strains.

5. Conclusion

The COVID-19 virus has continued to adapt and persist beyond 2020 and will likely continue in some form for years to come. Learning from the continued spread of this deadly virus is critical, and responses by governments to the global spread of COVID-19 has continuously adapted to new challenges and developing information. The consequences of the pandemic cannot be underestimated and has caused serious impacts on the global economy and healthcare capacity, as well as the physical and mental health of the public. COVID-19 associated morbidity and mortalities continue to climb across the world, even with the distribution of effective vaccines. Indeed, as travel restrictions are slowly lifted across the globe, the implementation of public health policies and expanding access to tracking the spread of the virus are powerful tools for minimizing unnecessary hospitalizations.

The world economy has suffered because of the pandemic, but only in part, as many countries enacted polices to prevent total recession, and some economies have even exhibited financial benefit. Specialized industries have yet to recover fully in 2022, and some businesses have been disproportionately impacted, owing to the challenges of public restrictions throughout 2020 and 2021. As major public restrictions begin to relax, many unrecovered industries can be expected to see continued economic improvements.

Having established efficient ways of tracking the COVID-19 virus through technological and biomolecular methods (e.g., nucleic acid amplification tests and WBE studies), governments around the world will be better prepared in surveying for future diseases of concern. Furthermore, with economists working on restructuring modern practices in supply-chain management, the world economies will be better prepared in the coming years to avoid similar challenges that are still prevalent two years into the pandemic.

Acknowledgements

This work was supported by the Saskatchewan Agricultural Development Fund (20190155, 20190154, 20180281, 20180248, 20180255, 20170133); National Sciences and Engineering Research Council of Canada Discovery Grant (RGPIN-2018-06631); and Mitacs (IT19122, IT16156).

Conflict of interest

Dr. Martin J. T. Reaney is the founder of, and has an equity interest in, Prairie Tide Diversified Inc. (PTD, Saskatoon, SK, Canada: previous company name is Prairie Tide Chemicals Inc.).

Author details

Timothy J. Tse*, Farley Chicilo*, Jeffrey Popiel* and Martin J.T. Reaney*
University of Saskatchewan, Saskatoon, Canada

*Address all correspondence to: timothy.tse@usask.ca; fhc246@mail.usask.ca; jeffrey.popiel@usask.ca and martin.reaney@usask.ca

References

[1] Loss Prevention Magazine. The Global Supply Chain Crisis: What Happened and When Will it End? [Internet]. 2022. Available from: https://losspreventionmedia.com/the-global-supply-chain-crisis/?msclkid=bf2bd13dc4c311ec9f713df83beb1b9f [Accessed: May 21, 2022]

[2] Hale T, Angrist N, Goldszmidt R, Kira B, Petherick A, Phillips T, et al. A global panel database of pandemic policies (Oxford COVID-19 government response tracker). Nature Human Behaviour. 2021;**5**:529-538. DOI: 10.1038/s41562-021-01079-8

[3] Klar R, Lanzerath D. The ethics of COVID-19 tracking apps – Challenges and voluntariness. Research Ethics. 2020;**16**: 1-9. DOI: 10.1177/1747016120943622

[4] Kondylakis H, Katehakis DG, Kouroubali A, Logothetidis F, Triantafyllidis A, Kalamaras I, et al. COVID-19 mobile apps: A systematic review of the literature. Journal of Medical Internet Research. 2020;**22**:e23170. DOI: 10.2196/23170

[5] Tangcharoensathien V, Bassett MT, Meng Q, Mills A. Are overwhelmed health systems an inevitable consequence of covid-19? Experiences from China, Thailand, and New York state. BMJ. 2021;**372**:n83. DOI: 10.1136/bmj.n83

[6] Mbunge E, Akinnuwesi B, Fashoto SG, Metfula AS, Mashwama P. A critical review of emerging technologies for tackling COVID-19 pandemic. Human Behavior and Emerging Technologies. 2021;**3**:25-39. DOI: 10.1002/hbe2.237

[7] Bartik A, Bertrand M, Cullen Z, Glaeser E, Luca M, Stanton C. The impact of COVID-19 on small business outcomes and expectations. Proceedings of the National Academy of Sciences. 2020;**117**:17656-17666. DOI: 10.1073/pnas.2006991117

[8] Tse TJ, Purdy SK, Shen J, Nelson FB, Mustafa R, Wiens DJ, et al. Toxicology of alcohol-based hand rubs formulated with technical-grade ethanol. Toxicology Reports. 2021;**8**:785-792. DOI: 10.1016/j.toxrep.2021.03.034

[9] Mustafa R, Purdy SK, Nelson FB, Tse TJ, Wiens DJ, Shen J, et al. Canadian policy changes for alcohol-based hand rubs during the COVID-19 pandemic and unintended risks. World med. Health Policy. 2021:1-13. DOI: 10.1002/wmh3.463

[10] Tse TJ, Nelson FB, Reaney MJT. Analyses of commercially available alcohol-based hand rubs formulated with compliant and non-compliant ethanol. International Journal of Environment Research. 2021;**18**:3766. DOI: 10.3390/ijerph18073766

[11] Reuters. Germany to Stop Free COVID-19 Tests – Report [Internet]. 2021. Available from: https://www.reuters.com/business/healthcare-pharmaceuticals/germany-stop-free-covid-19-tests-report-2021-08-09/ [Accessed: June 6, 2022]

[12] Farkas K, Hillary LS, Malham SK, McDonald JE, Jones DL. Wastewater and public health: The potential of wastewater surveillance for monitoring COVID-19. Current Opinion in Environmental Science & Health. 2020;**17**:14-20. DOI: 10.1016/j.coesh.2020.06.001

[13] Kirby AE, Walters MS, Jennings WC, Fugitt R, LaCross N, Mattioli M, et al.

Using wastewater surveillance data to support the COVID-19 response – United States, 2020-2021. MMWR. 2021;**70**:1242-1244. DOI: 10.15585/mmwr.mm7036a2

[14] Global Institute of Water Security. COVID-19 Early Indicators [Internet]. 2022. Available from https://water.usask.ca/covid-19/ [Accessed: April 8, 2022]

[15] Monteiro S, Rente D, Cunha MV, Gomes MC, Marques TA, Lourenço AB, et al. A wastewater-based epidemiology tool for COVID-19 surveillance in Portugal. Science of the Total Environment. 2022;**804**:150264. DOI: 10.1016/j.scitotenv.2021.150264

[16] Larsen DA, Wigginton KR. Tracking COVID-19 with wastewater. Nature Biotechnology. 2020;**38**:1151-1153. DOI: 10.1038/s41587-020-0690-1

[17] Rooney CM, Moura IB, Wilcox MH. Tracking COVID-19 via sewage. Current Opinion in Gastroenterology. 2021;**37**:4-8. DOI: 10.1097/MOG.0000000000000692

[18] Nghiem LD, Morgan B, Donner E, Short MD. The COVID-19 pandemic: Considerations for the waste and wastewater services sector. CSCEE. 2020;**1**:100006. DOI: 10.1016/j.cscee.2020.100006

[19] Berglund EZ, Thelemaque N, Spearing L, Faust KM, Kaminsky J, Sela L, et al. Water and wastewater systems and utilities: Challenges and opportunities during the COVID-19 pandemic. Journal of Water Resources Planning and Management. 2021;**147**:02521001

[20] Aguiar-Oliveira MDL, Campos AR, Matos A, Rigotto C, Sotero-Martins A, Teixeira PFP, et al. Wastewater-based epidemiology (WBE) and viral detection in polluted surface water: A valuable tool for COVID-19 surveillance – A brief review. International Journal of Environmental Research and Public Health. 2020;**17**:9251. DOI: 10.3390/ijerph17249251

[21] Ahmed W, Tscharke B, Bertsch PM, Bibby K, Bivins A, Choi P, et al. SARS-CoV-2 RNA monitoring in wastewater as a potential early warning system for COVID-19 transmission in the community: A temporal case study. Science of the Total Environment. 2021;**761**:14426. DOI: 10.1016/j.scitotenv.2020144216

[22] Gonzalez R, Curtis K, Bivins A, Bibby K, Weir MH, Yetka K, et al. COVID-19 surveillance in southeastern Virginia using wastewater-based epidemiology. Water Research. 2020;**186**:116296. DOI: 10.1016/j.watres.2020.116296

[23] Government of Canada. State of Trade 2021 – A Closer Look at Foreign Direct Investment (FDI) [Internet]. 2021. Available from: https://www.international.gc.ca/transparency-transparence/state-trade-commerce-international/2021.aspx [Accessed: May 21, 2022]

[24] Statistics Canada. Gross Domestic Product (GDP) at Basic Prices, by Industry, Monthly (x 1,000,000). 2022. Available from: https://www150.statcan.gc.ca/t1/tbl1/en/tv.action?pid=3610043401 [Accessed: June 3, 2022]

[25] Bureau of Economic Analysis. Gross Domestic Product (Third Estimate), Corporate Profits, and GDP by Industry, Fourth Quarter and Year 2021 [Internet]. 2022. Available from: https://www.bea.gov/sites/default/files/2022-03/gdp4q21_3rd.pdf [Accessed: May 26, 2022]

[26] The White House. Why the Pandemic Has Disrupted Supply Chains

[Internet]. 2021. Available from: https://www.whitehouse.gov/cea/written-materials/2021/06/17/why-the-pandemic-has-disrupted-supply-chains/ [Accessed: May 21, 2022]

[27] Seric A, Görg H, Liu W, Windisch M. Risk, Resilience, and Recalibration in Global Value Chains [Internet]. 2021. Available from: https://voxeu.org/article/risk-resilience-and-recalibration-global-value-chains [Accessed: June 3, 2022]

[28] Government of Canada. Technical-Grade Ethanol for use in hand Sanitizers and Hard-Surface Disinfectants: Notice to industry [Internet]. 2020. Available from: https://www.canada.ca/en/health-canada/services/drugs-health-products/natural-non-prescription/legislation-guidelines/covid19-technical-grade-ethanol-hand-sanitizer.html [Accessed: May 21, 2022]

[29] Government of Canada. Licensing Approach to Produce and Distribute alcohol-Based Hand Sanitizers: Guidance Document [Internet] 2020. Available from: https://www.canada.ca/en/health-canada/services/drugs-health-products/drug-products/applications-submissions/guidance-documents/covid-19-expediated-licensing-alcohol-hand-sanitizer.html [Accessed: May 21, 2022]

[30] Government of Canada. Expedited Access to Disinfectants, Hand Sanitizers and Personal Protective Equipment to Help Limit the Spread of COVID-19, as well as Swabs for Testing [Internet]. 2020. Available from: https://recalls-rappels.canada.ca/en/alert-recall/expedited-access-disinfectants-hand-sanitizers-and-personal-protective-equipment-help?msclkid=c2996cb7c4e311ec8a800161041e8606 [Accessed: May 21, 2022]

[31] International Labour Organization. Impact of the COVID-19 Crisis on Loss of Jobs and Hours Among Domestic Workers [Internet]. 2020. Available from: https://www.ilo.org/wcmsp5/groups/public/---ed_protect/---protrav/---travail/documents/publication/wcms_747961.pdf [Accessed: May 21, 2022]

[32] Ragan. Research: Key Factors Fueling 'The Great Resignation' [Internet]. 2021. Available from: https://www.ragan.com/research-key-factors-fueling-the-great-resignation/?msclkid=eb8c5cf5c4c911ec8da582649fb9537d [Accessed: May 21, 2022]

[33] Tessema M, Tesfom G, Faircloth M, Tesfagiorgis M, Teckle P. The "great resignation": Causes, consequences, and creative HR management strategies. Journal of Human Resource Sustainability Studies. 2022;**10**:161-178. DOI: 10.4236/jhrss.2022.101011

[34] United States International Trade Commission. The Impact of the COVID-19 Pandemic on Freight Transportation Services and U.S. Merchandise Imports [Internet]. 2020. Available from: https://www.usitc.gov/research_and_analysis/tradeshifts/2020/special_topic.html [Accessed: May 21, 2022]

[35] Supply Chains. Chemical Manufacturing Supply Chain [Internet]. 2021. Available from: https://comptroller.texas.gov/economy/economic-data/supply-chain/2021/chem.php [Accessed: May 21, 2022]

[36] OECD. Gross Domestic Product (GDP) (indicator) [Internet]. 2022. Available from: https://www.oecd-ilibrary.org/economics/gross-domestic-product-gdp/indicator/english_dc2f7aec-en [Accessed: June 6, 2022]

[37] OECD. Quarterly GDP (indicator) [Internet]. 2022. Available from: https://www.oecd-ilibrary.org/economics/quarterly-gdp/indicator/english_b86d1fc8-en [Accessed: June 3, 2022]

[38] Liu X, Ornelas E, Shi H. The 2020 Trade Impact of the COVID-19 Pandemic [Internet]. 2021. Available from: https://voxeu.org/article/2020-trade-impact-covid-19-pandemic [Accessed June 3, 2022]

[39] Arriola C, Kowalski P, van Tongeren F. Localising Value Chains in the post-COVID World Would add to the Economic Losses and Make Domestic Economies more Vulnerable [Internet]. 2020. Available from: https://voxeu.org/article/localising-value-chains-after-covid-would-add-economic-losses-and-make-domestic-economies-more-vulnerable [Accessed: June 3, 2022]

[40] Pisch F. Just-in-time Supply Chains after the COVID-19 Crisis. [Internet]. 2020. Available from: https://voxeu.org/article/just-time-supply-chains-after-covid-19-crisis [Accessed: June 3, 2022]

[41] Magableh GM. Supply chains and the COVID-19 pandemic: A comprehensive framework. European Management Review. 2021;**18**:363-382. DOI: 10.1111/emre.12449

[42] Thunström L, Newbold S, Finnoff D, Ashworth M, Shogren J. The benefits and costs of using social distancing to flatten the curve for COVID-19. Journal of Benefit-Cost Analysis. 2020;**11**:179-195. DOI: 10.1017/bca.2020.12

[43] Chan EYY, Huang Z, Lo ESK, Hung KKC, Wong ELY, Wong SYS. Sociodemographic predictors of health risk perception, attitude and behavior practices associated with health-emergency disaster risk Management for Biological Hazards: The case of COVID-19 pandemic in Hong Kong, SAR China. International Journal of Environmental Research and Public Health. 2020;**17**:3869. DOI: 10.3390/ijerph17113869

[44] Wells CR, Sah P, Moghadas SM, Pandey A, Shoukat A, Wang Y, et al. Impact of international travel and border control measures on the global spread of the novel 2019 coronavirus outbreak. Proceedings of the National Academy of Sciences. 2020;**117**:7504-7509. DOI: 10.1073/pnas.2002616117

[45] Mann DM, Chen J, Chunara R, Testa PA, Nov O. COVID-19 transforms health care through telemedicine: Evidence from the field. Journal of the American Medical Informatics Association. 2020;**27**:1132-1135. DOI: 10.1093/jamia/ocaa072

[46] Ritchie H, Mathieu E, Rodés-Guirao L, Appel C, Giattino C, Ortiz-Ospina E, Joe Hasell, Macdonald B, Beltekian D, and Roser M. Coronavirus Pandemic (COVID-19) [Internet]. 2020. Available from: https://ourworldindata.org/coronavirus [Accessed: May 15, 2022]

[47] Iyengar K, Bahl S, Vaishya R, Vaish A. Challenges and solutions in meeting up the urgent requirement of ventilators for COVID-19 patients. Diabetes and Metabolic Syndrome: Clinical Research and Reviews. 2020;**14**:499-450. DOI: 10.1016/j.dsx.2020.04.048

[48] Tyrrell CSB, Mytton OT, Gentry SV, Thomas-Meyer M, Allen JLY, Narula AA, et al. Managing intensive care admissions when there are not enough beds during the COVID-19 pandemic: A system review. Thorax. 2021;**76**:302-312. DOI: 10.1136/thoraxjnl-2020-215518

[49] Rasmussen S, Sperling P, Poulsen MS, Emmersen J, Andersen S. Medical students for health-care staff shortages during the COVID-19 pandemic. The Lancet. 2020;**395**:79-80. DOI: 10.1016/S0140-6736(20)30923-5

[50] Mulugeta T, Tadesse E, Shegute T, Desta T. COVID-19: Socio-economic

impacts and challenges in the working group. Heliyon. 2021;7:e07307. DOI: 10.1016/j.heliyon.2021.e07307

[51] Bick A, Blandin A, Mertens K. Work from home after the Covid-19 Outbreak [Internet]. 2021. Available from: https://www.dallasfed.org/-/media/documents/research/papers/2020/wp2017r1.pdf [Accessed: June 3, 2022]

[52] Shortall R, Mouter N, Van Wee B. COVID-19 and transport. A review of factors of relevance to the design of measures and their effects worldwide. European Journal of Transport and Infrastructure Research. 2022, 2020;**22**:118-130. DOI: 10.18757/ejtir.2022.22.1.5597

[53] Haider M, Anwar AI. The prevalence of telework under Covid-19 in Canada. Information Technology and People. 2022. DOI: 10.1108/ITP-08-2021-0585

[54] Prem K, Liu Y, Russell TW, Kucharski AJ, Eggo RM, Davies N, et al. The effect of control strategies to reduce social mixing on outcomes of the COVID-19 epidemic in Wuhan, China: A modelling study. The Lancet Public Health. 2020;**5**:261-270. DOI: 10.1016/S2468-2667(20)30073-6

[55] Gupta N, Rana S, Panda S, Bhargava B. Use of COVID-19 test positivity rate, epidemiological, and clinical tools for guiding targeted public health interventions. Frontiers in Public Health. 2022;**10**:821611-821611. DOI: 10.3389/fpubh.2022.821611

[56] Mahmoudi J, Xiong C. How social distancing, mobility, and preventive policies affect COVID-19 outcomes: Big data-driven evidence from the District of Columbia-Maryland-Virginia (DMV) megaregion. PLoS One. 2022;**17**:e0263820. DOI: 10.1371/journal.pone.0263820

[57] Huntley K, Wahood W, Mintz J, Raine S, Hardigan P, Haffizulla F. Associations of stay-at-home order enforcement with COVID-19 population outcomes: An interstate statistical analysis. American Journal of Epidemiology. 2022;**91**:561-569. DOI: 10.1093/aje/kwab267

[58] Burki T. Lifting of COVID-19 restrictions in the UK and the Delta variant. The Lancet Respiratory Medicine. 2021;**9**:e85. DOI: 10.1016/S2213-2600(21)00328-3

[59] Andal V, Lakshmipathy R, Jose D. Effect of sanitizer on obliteration of SARS –CoV2/COVID 19: A mini review. Materials Today: Proceedings. 2022;**55**:264-266. DOI: 10.1016/j.matpr.2021.07.026

[60] Government of Canada. (2020a). Hard-Surface Disinfectants and Hand Sanitizers (COVID-19): Disinfectants and Hand Sanitizers Accepted under COVID-19 Interim Measure [Internet]. 2021. Available from: https://www.canada.ca/en/health-canada/services/drugs-health-products/disinfectants/covid-19/products-accepted-under-interim-measure.html [Accessed: May 26, 2022]

[61] International Food & Agricultural Trade Policy Council. Agricultural Export Restrictions: Welfare Implications and Trade Disciplines [Internet]. 2009. Available from: https://www.researchgate.net/profile/Siddhartha-Mitra-5/publication/331478130_Agricultural_Export_Restrictions_Welfare_Implications_and_Trade_Disciplines/links/5c7bb80692851c69504f933d/Agricultural-Export-Restrictions-Welfare-Implications-and-Trade-Disciplines.pdf [Accessed: June 6, 2022]

[62] Strickland J, Reed D, Hursh S, Schwartz L, Foster R, Gelino B. Johnson, M behavioral economic methods to

inform infectious disease response: Prevention, testing, and vaccination in the COVID-19 pandemic. PLoS One. 2022;**17**:e0258828. DOI: 10.1371/journal.pone.0258828

[63] Mercer T, Salit M. Testing at scale during the COVID-19 pandemic. Nature Reviews. Genetics. 2021;**22**:415-426. DOI: 10.1038/s41576-021-00360-w

[64] Guan D, Wang D, Hallegatte S, Davis S, Huo J, Li S, et al. Global supply-chain effects of COVID-19 control measures. Nature Human Behaviour. 2020;**4**:577-587. DOI: 10.1038/s41562-020-0896-8

[65] Songok E. A locally sustainable approach to COVID-19 testing in Africa. The Lancet Microbe. 2020;**1**:e197. DOI: 10.1016/S2666-5247(20)30118-X

[66] Xing Y, Wong G, Ni W, Hu X, Xing Q. Rapid response to an outbreak in Qingdao, China. The New England Journal of Medicine. 2020;**383**:e129. DOI: 10.1056/NEJMc2032361

[67] Bateman AC, Mueller S, Guenther K, Shult P. Assessing the dilution effect of specimen pooling on the sensitivity of SARS-CoV-2 PCR tests. Journal of Medical Virology. 2020;**93**:1568-1572. DOI: 10.1002/jmv.26519

[68] Linkov I, Keenan JM, Trump BD, editors. COVID-19: Systemic Risk and Resilience. 1st ed. Cham: Springer; 2021. pp. 1-9. DOI: 10.1007/978-3-030-71587-8

[69] Garg S, Kim L, Whitaker M, O'Halloran A, Cummings C, Holstein R, et al. Hospitalization rates and characteristics of patients hospitalized with laboratory-confirmed coronavirus disease 2019 — Covid-net, 14 states, march 1-30, 2020. MMWR. 2020;**69**:458-464. DOI: 10.15585/mmwr.mm6915e3

[70] Hooper MW, Na'poles AM, Pe'rez-Stable EJ. COVID-19 and racial/ethnic disparities. Journal of the American Medical Association. 2020;**323**:2466-2467. DOI: 10.1001/jama.2020.8598

[71] Jin JM, Bai P, He W, Wu F, Liu XF, Han DM, et al. Gender differences in patients with COVID-19: Focus on severity and mortality. Frontiers in Public Health. 2020;**8**:152. DOI: 10.3389/fpubh.2020.00152

[72] Brodeur A, Gray D, Islam A, Bhuiyan S. A literature review of the economics of COVID-19. Journal of Economic Surveys. 2021;**35**:1007-1044. DOI: 10.1111/joes.12423

[73] Belot M, Choi S, Tripodi E, Broek-Altenburg E, Jamison J, Papageorge N. Unequal consequences of Covid 19: Representative evidence from six countries. Review of Economics of the Household. 2021;**19**:769-783. DOI: 10.1007/s11150-021-09560-z

[74] Maxwell H. COVID-19: A lonely pandemic. Cities & Health. 2020;**5**:S80-S82. DOI: 10.1080/23748834.2020.1788770

[75] Kalluri N, Kelly C, Garg A. Child care during the COVID-19 pandemic: A bad situation made worse. Pediatric. 2021;**147**:1. DOI: 10.1542/peds.2020-041525

[76] Piquero A, Jennings W, Jemison E, Kaukinen C, Knaul F. Domestic violence during the COVID-19 pandemic - evidence from a systematic review and meta-analysis. Journal of Criminal Justice. 2021;**74**:101806. DOI: 10.1016/j.jcrimjus.2021.101806

[77] Colbert S, Wilkinson C, Thornton L, Richmond R. COVID-19 and alcohol in Australia: Industry changes and public

health impacts. Drug and Alcohol Review. 2020;**39**:435-440. DOI: 10.1111/dar.13092

[78] Kola L, Kohrt B, Hanlon C, Naslund J, Sikander S, Balaji M, et al. COVID-19 mental health impact and responses in low-income and middle-income countries: Reimagining global mental health. Lancet Psychiatry. 2021;**8**:535-550. DOI: 10.1016/s2215-0366(21)00025-0

[79] Ciotti M, Ciccozzi M, Pieri M, Bernardini S. The COVID-19 pandemic: Viral variants and vaccine efficacy. Critical Reviews in Clinical Laboratory Sciences. 2022;**59**:66-75. DOI: 10.1080/10408363.2021.1979462

[80] Sallam M. COVID-19 vaccine hesitancy worldwide: A concise systematic review of vaccine acceptance rates. Vaccine. 2021;**9**:160. DOI: 10.3390/vaccines9020160

[81] Williams SN, Armitage CJ, Tampe T, Dienes K. Public attitudes towards COVID-19 contact tracing apps: A UK-based focus group study. Health Expectations. 2021;**24**:377-385. DOI: 10.1111/hex.13179

[82] Ferretti L, Wymant C, Kendall M, Zhao L, Nurtay A, Abeler-Dörner L, et al. Quantifying SARS-CoV-2 transmission suggests epidemic control with digital contact tracing. Science. 2020;**368**:eabb6936. DOI: 10.1126/science.abb6936

[83] Government of Canada. Download COVID Alert Today. [Internet]. 2021. Available from https://www.canada.ca/en/public-health/services/diseases/coronavirus-disease-covid-19/covid-alert.html [Accessed: April 10, 2022]

[84] Rimmer A. Sixty seconds on . . . The pingdemic. BMJ. 2021;**374**:n1822. DOI: 10.1136/bmj.n1822

[85] CTV News. Wastewater Now 'One of Our Only Reliable Tools' to Detect COVID-19 Prevalence. [Internet]. 2022. Available from: https://www.ctvnews.ca/health/coronavirus/wastewater-now-one-of-our-only-reliable-tools-to-detect-covid-19-prevalence-1.5862546 [Accessed: April 16, 2022]

[86] Rangaiah A, Shankar SM, Basawarajappa SG, Shah PA, Chandrashekar A, Munegowda A, et al. Detection of SARS-CoV-2 in clinical samples: Target-specific analysis of qualitative reverse transcription-polymerase chain reaction (RT-PCR) diagnostic kits. IJID Regions. 2021;**1**:163-169. DOI: 10.1016/j.ijregi.2021.11.004

[87] Agrawal S, Orschler L, Lackner S. Long-term monitoring in SARS-CoV-2 RNA in wastewater of the Frankfurt metropolitan of area in southern Germany. Scientific Reports. 2021;**11**:5372. DOI: 10.1038/s41598-021-84914-2

[88] van Kasteren PB, van der Veer B, van den Brink S, Wijsman L, de Jonge J, van den Brandt A, et al. Comparison of seven commercial RT-PCR diagnostic kits for COVID-19. Journal of Clinical Virology. 2020;**128**:104412. DOI: 10.1016/j.jcv.2020.104412

[89] National Center for Biotechnology Information (NCBI). ORF1ab polyprotein [Severe acute respiratory syndrome coronavirus 2] [Internet]. 2022. Available from: https://www.ncbi.nlm.nih.gov/gene/43740578 [Accessed: April 18, 2022]

[90] Kirtipal N, Bharadwaj S, Kang SG. From SARS to SARS-COV-2, insights on structure, pathogenicity and immunity aspects of pandemic human coronaviruses. Infection, Genetics and Evolution. 2020;**85**:104502. DOI: 10.1016/j.meegid.2020.104502

[91] Barreto HG, de Pàdua Milagres FA, de Araújo GC, Daúde MM, Benedito VA. Diagnosing the novel SARS-CoV-2 by quantitative RT-PCR: Variations and opportunities. Journal of Molecular Medicine. 2020;**98**:1727-1736. DOI: 10.1007/s00109-020-01992-x

[92] Lu X, Wang L, Sakthivel SK, Whitaker B, Murray J, Kamili S, et al. US CDC real-time reverse transcription PCR panel for detection of severe acute respiratory syndrome coronavirus 2. Emerging Infectious Diseases. 2020;**26**:1654-1665. DOI: 10.3201/eid2608.201246

[93] Daughton C. The international imperative to rapidly and inexpensively monitor community-wide COVID-19 infection status and trends. Science of the Total Environment. 2020;**726**:138149. DOI: 10.1016/j.scitotenv.2020.138149

[94] Sinclair RG, Choi CY, Riley MR, Gerba CP. Pathogen surveillance through monitoring of sewer systems. Advances in Applied Microbiology. 2008;**65**:249-269. DOI: 10.1016/S0065-2164(08)00609-6

[95] Centers for Disease Control and Prevention. Nucleic Acid Amplification Tests (NAATs). [Internet]. 2022. Available from: https://www.cdc.gov/coronavirus/2019-ncov/lab/naats.html#:~:text=The_NAAT_procedure_works_by,sensitive_for_diagnosing_COVID_19 [Accessed: April 8, 2022]

[96] Ghernaout D, Ghernaout B. Controlling COVID-19 pandemic through wastewater monitoring. OALib Journal. 2020;**7**:e6411. DOI: 10.4236/oalib.1106411

[97] Saththasivam J, El-Malah SS, Gomez TA, Jabbar KA, Remanan R, Krishnankutty AK, et al. COVID-19 (SARS-CoV-2) outbreak monitoring using wastewater-based epidemiology in Qatar. Science of the Total Environment. 2021;**774**:145608. DOI: 10.1016/j.scitotenv.2021.145608

[98] Haramoto E, Kitajima M, Hata A, Torrey JR, Masago Y, Sano D, et al. A review on recent progress in the detection methods and prevalence of human enteric viruses in water. Water Research. 2018;**135**:168-186. DOI: 10.1016/j.watres.2018.02.004

[99] Bofill-Mas S, Rusiñol M. Recent trends on methods for the concentration of viruses from water samples. Current Opinion in Environmental Science Health. 2020;**16**:7-13. DOI: 10.1016/j.coesh.2020.01.006

[100] Wurtzer S, Marechal V, Mouchel JM, Maday Y, Teyssou R, Richard E, et al. Evaluation of lockdown effect on SARS-CoV-2 dynamics through viral genome quantification in waste water, greater Paris, France, 5 march to 23 April 2020. Euro Surveillance. 2020;**25**:2000776. DOI: 10.2807/1560-7917.ES.2020.25.50.2000776

[101] Ahmed W, Angel N, Edson J, Bibby K, Bivins A, O'Brien JW, et al. First confirmed detection of SARS-CoV-2 in untreated wastewater in Australia: A proof of concept for the wastewater surveillance of COVID-19 in the community. Science of the Total Environment. 2020;**728**:138764. DOI: 10.1016/j.scitotenv.2020.138764

[102] Medema G, Heijnen L, Elsinga G, Italiaander R, Brouwer A. Presence of SARS-Coronavirus-2 RNA in sewage and correlation with reported COVID-19 prevalnce in the early stage of the epidemic in the Netherlands. Environmental Science & Technology Letters. 2020;**7**:511-516. DOI: 10.1021/acs.estlett.0c00357

[103] Bar-Or I, Yaniv K, Shagan M, Ozer E, Weil M, Indenbaum V, et al. Regressing SARS-CoV-2 sewage measurements onto COVID-19 burden in the population:

A proof-of-concept for quantitative environmental surveillance. Frontiers in Public Health. 2021;**9**:561710. DOI: 10.3389/fpubh.2021.561710

[104] Nemudri A, Nemudraia A, Wiegand T, Surya K, Buyukyoruk M, Cicha C, et al. Temporal detection and phylogenetic assessment of SARS-CoV-2 in municipal wastewater. Cell Reports. 2020;**1**:100098. DOI: 10.1016/j.xcrm.2020.100098

[105] Balboa S, Mauricio-Iglesias M, Rodríguez S, Martínez-Lamas L, Vasallo FJ, Regueiro B, et al. The fate of SARS-CoV-2 in WWTPS points out the sludge line as a suitable spot for detection of COVID-19. Science of the Total Environment. 2021;**772**:145268. DOI: 10.1016/j.scitotenv.2021.145268

[106] Wu F, Zhang J, Xiao A, Gu X, Lee WL, Armas F, et al. SARS-CoV-2 titers in wastewater are higher than expected from clinically confirmed cases. mSystems. 2020;**5**:e00614-e00620. DOI: 10.1128/msystems.00614-20

[107] Zhang D, Ling H, Huang X, Li J, Li W, Yi C, et al. Potential spreading risks and disinfection challenges of medical wastewater by the presence of severe acute respiratory syndrome coronavirus 2 (SARS-CoV-2). Science of the Total Environment. 2020;**741**:140445. DOI: 10.1016/j.scitotenv.2020.140445

[108] Randazzo W, Cuevas-Ferrando E, Sanjuán R, Domingo-Calap P, Sánchez G. Metropolitan wastewater analysis for COVID-19 epidemiological survey. International Journal of Hygiene and Environmental Health. 2020;**230**:113621. DOI: 10.1016/j.ijheh.2020.113621

[109] Randazzo W, Truchado P, Cuevas-Ferrando E, Simón P, Allende A, Sánchez G. SARS-CoV-2 RNA in wastewater anticipated COVID-19 occurrence in a low prevalence area. Water Research. 2020;**181**:115942. DOI: 10.1016/j.watres.2020.115942

[110] Bisseux M, Didier D, Audrey M, Christine A, Hélène PL, Jean-Luc B, et al. Monitoring of enterovirus diversity in wastewater by ultra-deep sequencing: An effective complementary tool for clinical enterovirus surveillance. Water Research. 2020;**169**:115246. DOI: 10.1016/j.watres.2019.115246

[111] Lun JH, Crosbie ND, White PA. Genetic diversity and quantification of human mastadenoviruses in wastewater from Sydney and Melbourne, Australia. Science of the Total Environment. 2019;**675**:305-312. DOI: 10.1016/j.scitotenv.2019.04.162

[112] Bibby K, Crank K, Greaves J, Li X, Wu Z, Hamza IA, et al. Metagenomics and the development of viral water quality tools. npj Clean Water. 2019;**2**:1-13. DOI: 10.1038/s41545-019-0032-3

[113] Miura T, Lhomme S, Le Saux JC, Le Mehaute P, Guillois Y, Couturier E, et al. Detection of hepatitis E virus in sewage after an outbreak on a French island. Food Environment Virology. 2016;**8**:194-199. DOI: 10.1007/s12560-016-9241-9

[114] Hata A, Katayama H, Kojima K, Sano S, Kasuga I, Kitajima M, et al. Effects of rainfall events on the occurrence and detection efficiency of viruses in river water impacted by combined sewer overflows. Science of the Total Environment. 2014;**268-269**:757-763. DOI: 10.1016/j.scitotenv.2013.08.093

[115] Bogler A, Packman A, Furman A, Gross A, Kushmaro A, Ronen A, et al. Rethinking wastewater risks and monitoring in light of the COVID-19 pandemic. Nature Sustainability. 2020;**3**:981-990. DOI: 10.1038/s41893-020-00605-2

Chapter 5

Zoonotic Parasites and Vector-Borne Parasitoses

Jasmin Omeragic, Sabina Seric-Haracic and Naida Kapo

Abstract

Zoonotic parasites and vector-borne zoonotic parasitoses of humans, especially when affecting immunocompromised persons mobilize researchers' interest and increase parasitological, environmental, and interdisciplinary investigations worldwide. Climate, environmental and anthropomorphic influences had affected the distribution, occurrence, and adaptability of parasites in humans and animals, the level of environmental contamination with parasites and their developing forms, and the surge of vector competency. Knowledge of parasite biology and evolution shows that hybridization phenomena and adaptations may cause genetic diversity, affecting parasite virulence, antiparasitic drug resistance, acclimatization to new host species, and environmental conditions previously not recorded while leading to the emergence of new diseases and changing parasitism epidemiology. Many parasitic infections are emerging or re-emerging and are neglected with deliberating consequences for public and animal health as well as for food safety and security, especially in sub capacitated developing countries. Decrease of exposure of both animals and humans and negative consequences of zoonotic parasitoses requires raising awareness of researchers, policymakers, and the wider public. Modern diagnostic methods, surveillance, monitoring of parasitoses, and early detection systems followed by tailored containment and control actions provide grounds for sane assessments and investigation toward the cost-effective and efficient prevention programs for both human and animal populations.

Keywords: parasitic zoonoses, vector-borne parasitoses, prevention, control

1. Introduction

Parasitism is defined as when one organism (parasite) lives on or within another (host) in close biological and ecological dependence, lasting for a certain period of the parasite life cycle. Zoonotic parasites represent particular parasites to whom mainly animals are hosts, but can as well infect and cause disease in humans. To maintain a parasitic relationship with a host, parasites adapted in different ways as part of their evolutionary development parallel to the phylogenetic development of their hosts. Parasites are recognized for many species of hosts, including plants, vertebrates, and invertebrates, with currently rising concerns of hybridization phenomena as a threat to public health, still not fully understood. The risk posed by hybridization and introgression is recognized based on the biology and evolution of parasites, where resulting adaptations may bring significant genetic diversity, affecting parasite virulence, antiparasitic drug resistance, acclimatization to new host species, and environmental conditions previously not recorded while leading to the emergence of new diseases and changing of parasitism epidemiology. Also, research of parasitoses, particularly zoonotic and vector-borne, gains attention in light of enhanced emergence and re-emergence of pathogens affecting humans and animals where many represent a serious threat to the host's health and wellbeing [1, 2].

As shown in **Figure 1** this is primarily caused by anthropogenic influences and continuous modifications of the environment (climate changes, deforestation, disturbance of ecosystems, etc.), practices of food production and consumption (intensive vs. traditional agriculture, global animal movement, and trade), socio-demographic changes and globalization (population growth, urbanization, international trade, tourism, and transportation). Accordingly, our research aimed to provide an overview of the current trends regarding globally most important zoonotic parasites, diseases they cause, and associated influence factors.

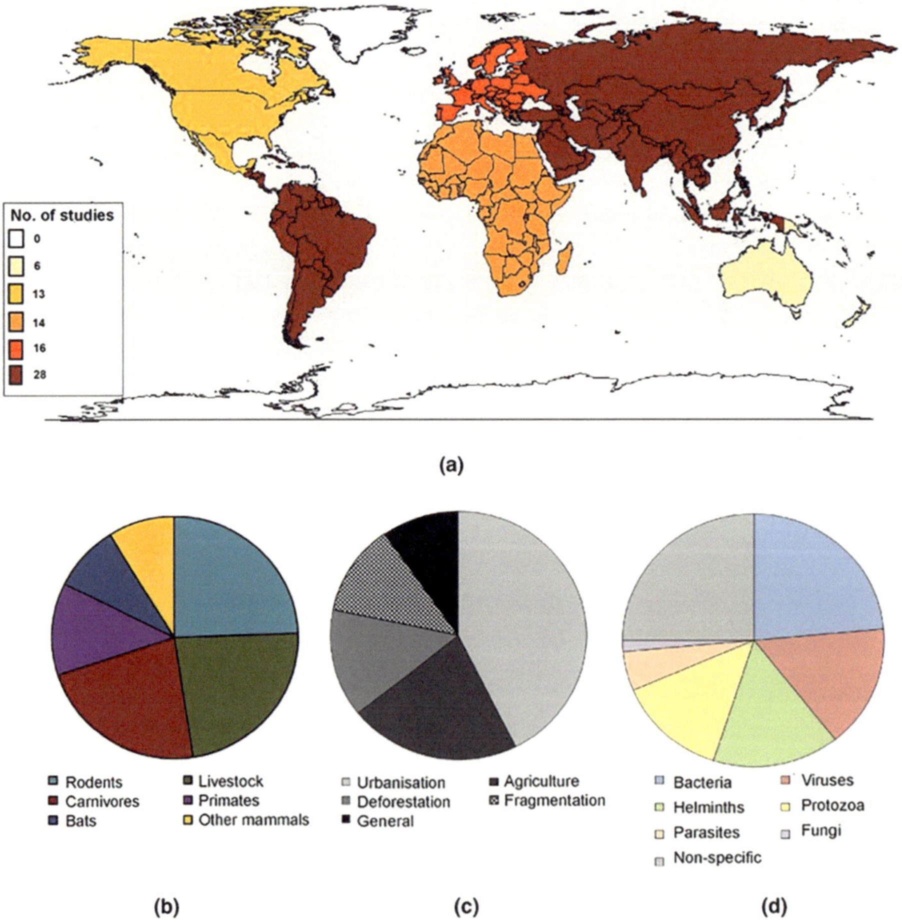

Figure 1.
Published research on mammalian zoonoses; color-coded based on geographic region (a), proportional frequency of papers dealing with different hosts (b), different anthropogenic influences (c), and different pathogens (d) [3].

Globalization and global warming in the twenty-first-century increase probability of parasitic infections in humans and animals and enable the introduction of most zoonotic parasites in new biotopes thus increasing the risk of epidemics occurrence in different areas [4]. Attempts to control parasitoses by mass treatment or vaccination are changing the environments in which parasites and other pathogens evolve, adapt, or extinct. Advances in diagnostics, especially molecular methods enable better recognition and characterization of pathogens hence improving outbreak detection and predictions. Continuous monitoring of parasites, vectors, hosts, and natural habitats in endemic areas, as well as early recognition systems, provide grounds for sound and timely epidemiological assessment and investigation leading to cost-effective and efficient prevention programs for parasitoses in both human and animal populations.

2. Methodology

Research inputs were identified through bibliographic database search using keywords: "zoonoses", "zoonotic pathogens", "zoonotic parasitoses", and "zoonotic parasites". In the first run, we excluded case/case series reports, clinical trials (assessment of treatment), and test validation (assessment of diagnostics), as well as a publication based on narrow geographical area, specific pathogen, disease, or hosts. Inclusion criteria for publications were prioritized based on the type of publication (first considered were review papers and global reports) and the topic/subject of a publication (publications reporting and exploring trends, global influences, and epidemiology). More recent publications covering wider geographical areas and multidisciplinary approaches or by author's affiliations were further considered. The selected literature review was oriented toward compiling and summarizing data on causative agents, distribution, life cycle, hosts, pathogenesis, symptoms, diagnostics, and therapy/treatment.

3. Zoonotic parasitoses in humans and animals

Numerous parasites found in animals, which represent final or intermediate hosts or vectors, are zoonotic or potentially zoonotic thus representing health risks for humans. In addition to direct and vector-borne transmission, an important source of human infections is the contaminated environment (i.e., geo-parasites, waterborne parasitoses), while some zoonotic parasites are foodborne. The majority of the common parasitic diseases of animals caused by helminths, trematodes, cestodes, pentastomids, and protozoa are zoonotic or have zoonotic potential. *Toxoplasma gondii* is the most widespread protozoan parasite worldwide. Estimates are that approximately one-third of the world's population is affected [5]. In developed countries, parasitic water-borne protozoans such as Cryptosporidium and Giardia outbreaks are increasingly reported [6]. In addition to protozoan parasites, the FAO identified *Taenia solium*, *Echinococcus granulosus*, *Echinococcus multilocularis*, Trichinella, Opisthorchiidae, and Ascaris spp. as the main foodborne parasites [7]. Data show that 70% of the helminths population is hosted by 15% of the host population, and these individuals are a prime source of environmental contamination [8]. The tapeworm *T. solium* is a cosmopolitan parasite with global distribution, with most human cases found in Latin America, Asia, and Africa alongside emergence in recent years in the USA and Europe [9]. In addition to widespread *E. granulosus*, recently *E. multilocularis* has become very important because of its expansion from endemic areas to non-endemic areas in North America, Europe, and Japan, apparently by a displacement of fox populations [10]. Regarding Trichinella spp., during the period 1986–2010, 65,818 new cases were registered in 41 countries. Of these, 87% occurred in Europe associated with boar consumption [10]. Characteristics of selected, most important zoonotic parasitoses are shown in **Table 1**.

Disease	Causative agent	Intermediate host	Hosts	Transmission	Distribution
Fascioliasis	Fasciola hepatica F. gigantica	Lymnaeid snails	Ruminants, horses, and pigs	Water and water plants	Parts of Europe, Middle East, Latin America, Caribbean, Asia, and Africa
Schistosomiasis	Schistosoma spp.	Freshwater snails	Various animals	Water (percutaneous penetration)	Africa, South America, Caribbean, Central, and West Africa, South-East Asia, and sub-Saharan Africa
Cystic echinococcosis	Echinococcus spp.	Sheep, cattle, moose, wallabies, camels, warthogs, reindeer, and pig	Carnivores (mainly dogs)	Water and food	Worldwide
Alveolar echinococcosis	Echinococcus multiocularis E. vogeli E. oligarthrus	Rodents	Carnivores, (red fox and dogs)	Water and food	Northern hemisphere
Taeniasis	Taenia spp.	Ruminants, pigs, rodents	Humans	Undercooked meat	Worldwide
Hymenolepiasis	*Hymenolepis nana* *H. diminuta*	Arthropods	Rodents and humans	Water and food	Worldwide
Trichinellosis	Trichinella spp.	Many vertebrate hosts	Various animals	Animal tissues	Worldwide
Toxocariasis and other geo-helminthiases	*Toxocara canis* *T. cati* Ascaris spp. Ancylostoma spp. *Uncinaria stenocephala* Trichuris spp. *Strongyloides stercoralis*	Birds, cats, prairie dogs, rabbits, rodents, pigs, and other		Water, food, soil	Worldwide

DOI: http://dx.doi.org/10.5772/intechopen.105120

Disease	Causative agent	Intermediate host	Hosts	Transmission	Distribution
Dirofilariosis	Dirofilaria spp.	Mosquitoes	Domestic dogs, coyotes, jackals, wolves, domestic cats, bobcats, ferrets, and foxes	Mosquitos	North and South America, Australia, Japan, and Europe
Capillariasis	*Capillaria hepatica* *C. the Philippines*	Rodents, wild and domestic carnivores' lagomorphs, swine, primates, fish	Humans, birds	Water and food	Thailand, and sporadic cases in other East and Southeast Asia
Trypanosomiasis	*Trypanosoma cruzi* *T. brucei rhodesiense* *T. brucei gambiense*	Invertebrate vector	Domestic pigs and cats, wildlife reservoirs include opossums, armadillos, raccoons, and woodrats	Kissing bugs	Mexico, Central, and South America
Leishmaniasis	Leishmania spp.	Sandflies	Cats, dogs, horses, and bats	Sand fly's	Visceral leishmaniasis -Bangladesh, Ethiopia, India, Nepal, South Sudan, Sudan, and Brazil. Cutaneous leishmaniasis - South and Central America, the Middle East, and Central Asia
Giardiasis	Giardia spp.	Dogs, cats, ruminants, and pigs		Water, food, and surfaces	Worldwide
Zoonotic malaria	*Plasmodium spp.*	Anopheles mosquitoes	Wild macaque, chimpanzee, humans	Anopheles mosquitos	South Sahara and parts of Oceania
Toxoplasmosis	Toxoplasma gondii	Pigs, ruminants, poultry, and rabbits	Cats	Water and food	Worldwide except in South America
Cryptosporidiosis	Cryptosporidium spp.	Cattle, sheep, pigs, goats, horses, and deer		Water and food	Worldwide
Babesiosis	Babesia spp.	Tick	Rodents, and ruminants	Ticks	Worldwide
Amebiasis	*Entamoeba hitolytica*	Mammals		Water and food	Worldwide

Table 1.
Zoonotic parasitoses of humans including disease, causative agent, intermediate/definitive host(s), transmission, and distribution.

Fascioliasis is caused by parasites of the genus *Fasciola*. In animals, the disease leads to significant economic losses, especially in sheep and cattle farming. Until 1990 it was considered a secondary important disease, however, in the last three decades is on the list of Neglected tropical diseases (NTDs) due to increased incidence of human infections [11]. Adults of *F. hepatica* and *F. gigantica* are found in the liver and biliary system of ruminants, equids, and other herbivores, while humans are accidental hosts for both species. *Fasciola* development starts with eggs excreted in the faces of infected animals that come in contact with fresh water. Miracidia developed from eggs penetrating intermediate host; freshwater snail were through stages of sporocysts, cercaria exit snails and encysts on water plants developing into infectious metacercaria. Ingested by the final host they reach adult form and penetrate through the intestinal wall in the abdomen where they attach to the liver. Estimates are that worldwide between 2.4 and 17 million humans are infected [12]. In humans, an acute form of the disease is manifested by symptoms when parasites migrate through the abdominal cavity toward the liver. Symptoms of the acute and chronic phases of the disease include fever, weakness, abdominal pain, and hepatomegaly. Diagnosis is by direct parasitological or indirect serological tests (i.e., ELISA), magnetic resonance, ultrasound, and computerized tomography. Most people are treated successfully with triclabendazole, even though increased resistance of liver flukes to triclabendazole represents a threat to successful therapy and disease control in endemic areas.

Schistosomiasis is NTD, caused by a fluke of the genus *Schistosoma*. At least five species can infect humans out of which the most important are *S. mansoni*, *S. haematobium,* and *S. japonicum*. Estimates are that currently over 290.8 million people are infected by these parasites, while 779 million are potentially exposed. The disease has a high case fatality rate with 280.000 fatal outcomes and 3.3 million cases with permanently affected health as a consequence of the disease. The largest number of cases is found in areas of sub-Saharan Africa, the Middle East, India, China, Brazil, the Philippines, and Venezuela. In 2013, the disease is confirmed in Corsica. The occurrence and transmission of schistosomiasis are usually related to poor living and sanitary conditions [13]. The life cycle of the parasite starts with excreting eggs found in faces and urine into water. Asexual reproduction of shistoma evolves in snails until the stage of the cercaria, which through water penetrate through the skin into the venous system of the hosts, and parasite in different tissues depending on the species. The S. *hematobium* is found in the bladder and urinary system, *S. japonicum* in the small intestines, and *S. mansoni* parasites in both small and large intestines. Acute schistosomiasis is followed by fever, dermatitis, headache, myalgia, and respiratory symptoms. Infections by the *S. hematobium* are manifested by dysuria and hematuria due to injuries to reproductive organs alongside increased inclination of hosts to other infections. Infections by the *S. japonicum* and *S. mansoni* show symptoms of hematochezia, diarrhea, and obstipation, with ulceration, fibrosis, and hyperplasia of affected tissues in the chronic form of the disease [13]. If the parasite comes to the central nervous system, neuroshistomiasis as the most severe form of the disease develops with granulomatosis lesions of the brain leading to epileptic caesuras, encephalopathies, damaged sight, and ataxia. Diagnosis of schistosomiasis is by confirmation of eggs in feces and urine, by tests such as ELISA and PCR, together with diagnostic imaging techniques. Prevention of schistosomiasis includes snail population control and improvement of sanitary conditions. The vaccine is still unavailable, while praziquantel is used for treatment, efficient only for fully undeveloped forms of the parasite in migrating phase within the host organism.

Opisthorchiasis and clonorchiasis are diseases caused by species of the family Opisthorchiidae, most commonly by *Opistorchis felineus*, *O. viverrini*, and *Clonorchis sinensis*. The life cycle includes intermediate hosts (freshwater snails and cyprinid fish), while final hosts are humans, cats, dogs, pigs, rats, birds, and fish. Eggs excreted by faces develop through stages of sporocyst, redia, and cercaria, which leave snails to infect fish and become metacercaria. The life cycle ends with the consummation of infected fish by final hosts (raw or undercooked), and metacercaria migrates into biliary ducts, sack, and liver [14]. Currently, 45 million people throughout Europe and Asia are infected with 700 million potentially exposed. Even though estimates vary, clonorchiasis prevalence continues to grow compared to figures in 1990ties, especially in China. Data show that the prevalence in dogs and cats is high (0.8–48.5% and up to 64.1%, respectively). Mild forms of opisthorchiasis and clonorchiasis have nonspecific symptoms including eosinophilia and cholestasis. Chronic disease in humans may be accompanied by cholangiocarcinoma. Diagnosis is by parasitological tests through detection of eggs in host feces, serological tests, and molecular methods. Treatment with praziquantel is very efficient (90–95%), with still no evidence of resistance development.

Cystic and alveolar echinococcosis is caused by larval forms of tapeworms of the genus *Echinococcus* and it is considered one of the most important parasitic diseases in the world. *E. granulosus* s.l. and s.s., *E. ortleppi*, *E. canadensis,* and *E. intermedius* cause cystic echinococcosis (CE). *E. multiocularis* causes alveolar echinococcosis (AE), as well as in rare cases *E. vogelii* and *E. oligarthus* [15]. Most frequently final hosts for *E. granulosus* are dogs and wild Canidae, with ruminants, horses, and pigs as intermediate hosts. Humans can be an intermediate host for both species, infected most commonly by eggs. In 98% of cases, parasite inhabits the liver where cysts are developed. The WHO considers AE as the first of 20 foodborne NTDs, while *E. multiocularis* takes third place. Adult forms of the parasite inhabit the small intestines of the final host with eggs excreted by feces and consumed by intermediate hosts. Through stages of protoscolex, the cestode becomes infectious with the final stage of the cycle represented by the consumption of infected tissues of intermediate hosts by the final host [9]. The AE occurs exclusively in the northern hemisphere. An increase in prevalence is related to the growth of the fox population, especially in periurban areas. The global burden of disease is estimated to be 18.200 new cases annually, out of which 1.600 cases are reported in Europe [9]. The CE is distributed worldwide in both humans and animals, representing a serious threat, especially in the Mediterranean, South America, and Central Asia. The CE and AE are chronic and severe diseases most commonly affecting the liver. The *E. multilocularis* forms multilocular cysts, while *E. granulosus* forms one hydatid cyst. The *E. granulosus* cysts manifest in clinical symptoms correlated with their size and pressure on nearby organs. The prognosis for the CE depends on the parasite location most commonly in the liver or lungs, while 20% of infections are located in the spleen, peritoneum, kidneys, bones, and sometimes brain and spinal cord. Diagnosis in final hosts is by parasitological, serological, and molecular tests. Postmortem examination of small intestines is considered the "gold standard" test because it confirms the presence and enables the identification of the parasite species. In humans' diagnosis is by imaging techniques, serological tests, and by histopathological examination. Benzimidazole is the sole appropriate therapy for the CE, while the AE treatment is by surgery, with limited success due to difficulties in the removal of parasitic cysts. Unfortunately, surgery can be performed only in 20–50% of cases, while in rest treatment is not recommended especially for chronic cases due to developed mass of the parasitic cysts and frequent metastasis of cysts into various other organs.

Hymenolepiasis is caused by cestode; *Hymenolepis nana* and H. *diminuta*, are distributed worldwide with endemic areas in parts of Asia, and central Europe. Central and South America and Africa. The disease is common in children living in poor hygiene and sanitary conditions, wherein some poor community's prevalence can reach up to 58%. Epidemiolocal data show around 175 million people are infected throughout the world [16]. The disease commonly is asymptomatic, while in some cases symptoms such as chronic diarrhea, abdominal pain, anorexia, itching, and slow growth in children are recorded. Infections by the *H. nana* and *H. diminuta* in the final stages develop into severe clinical forms, sometimes life-threatening, especially in people with AIDS. The *H. nana* parasites in rodents, with direct human to human transmission and autoinfections. However, infection by the *H. nana* is still considered zoonotic due to widespread infections in rodents which serve as pathogen reservoirs. Humans can pose both intermediate and final hosts, while in the zoonotic transmission cycle arthropods have the role of intermediate hosts found in flour and grain. Accidental consumption of infected arthropods leads to the development of parasitic worms in humans. Diagnosis is made by confirmation of eggs in feces, while treatment includes praziquantel, nitazoxanide, and nicodamids.

Taeniasis is caused by the parasites of the genus *Taenia*. Species infecting humans are *Taenia solium* (pig tapeworm), *Taenia saginata* (cattle tapeworm), and *Taenia asiatica* (Asia tapeworm). Taeniasis is endemic in some developing countries, especially in Africa, South America, and Asia [17]. In countries of North America and Australia, disease occurs due to an increase in pig meat consumption, migrations, and travel. In epidemic form, taeniasis occurs in Spain and Portugal and sporadically in other countries of Western Europe. People are infected through consumption of undercooked pig or beef meat infected by the development form of the parasite (cysticercus), with the final location of the adult parasite in the small intestines. Also, in cases of feco-oral ingestion of *T. solium* eggs, the cysticercus develops in the human body causing neurocysticercosis (NCC) if development occurs in the central nervous system. The NCC is the most common form of taeniasis and raises great concerns in endemic areas. It causes about 50.000 death annually, and it is considered the most common cause of acquired epilepsy with about 2 million infections worldwide [17]. The symptoms are non-specific and include loss of weight, abdominal pain, vomiting, diarrhea, and obstipation. The symptoms of the NCC depend on the size, number, and location of cysts. The most common symptom of the NCC is epilepsy, followed by remittent headache due to increased intracranial pressure. If cysts are located in chambers of the brain, obstruction of cerebrospinal fluid flow causes hydrocephalus. Diagnosis is by parasitological, serological (ELISA), and molecular (PCR) methods. Albendazole and praziquantel are the most common antiparasitic drugs applied.

Trichinellosis is caused by the parasite of the genus *Trichinella*, transmitted through the consumption of raw or undercooked meat containing larva forms of the parasite [18]. There are at least 13 species/genotypes of Trichinella divided into two groups: incapsulated (*Trichinella spiralis*, *T. nativa*, *T. britovi*, *T. nelsoni*, *T. murelli*, and *T. pathogenesis*, *T. chanchalensis*, T6, T7, T8, and T9) and unencapsulated (*T. pseudospiralis*, *T. papuae*, *T. zimbawensis*). The life cycle starts with the enteric phase after larval ingestion (L1), which after several stages develop within 1–2 days in adult forms. After 30 h post-infection parasite starts to reproduce and newborn larvae start the parenteral phase by penetrating lymphatic and vascular systems. After reaching well-vascularized tissues, (skeletal muscles, myocardium, extraocular and intercostal muscles, and brain) they continue postembryonic development. Trichinellosis even though long known is still widely reported due to disturbances in the ecosystems caused by humans, where trichinella had successfully adapted and infects wild and domesticated animals, and humans in Eastern Europe, Asia, and South America [18]. Diagnosis is based on clinical examination, blood analysis (eosinophilia and increase in muscle enzyme levels), and epidemiological data. Direct diagnosis is made by PCR, digestion test, and histological examination of tissues collected by biopsy. Indirect diagnostic techniques include serological tests. Antiparasitic treatment includes benzimidazole, mostly albendazole with high therapeutic efficacy. Other antiparasitics such as ivermectin, nitazoxanide, quinfamide, and flubendazole are also good treatment alternatives.

4. Toxocariasis and other soil-transmitted helminthiases

Toxocariasis is a widely distributed zoonosis with a huge socio-economic impact, especially in poor countries. The disease is caused by the nematode of the genus *Toxocara*, which includes four species; *Toxocara canis*, *T. cati*, *T. malaysiensis,* and *T. vitulorum* able to infect a wide host range. Species *T. canis*, *T. cati,* and *T. malaysiensis* are common parasites of dogs, cats, and other carnivores with importance in veterinary and public health [19]. Toxocariasis in humans is manifested in four main clinical forms: visceral larva migrans, asymptomatic or common toxocariasis, and ocular and neuro-toxocariasis. The largest number of ocular toxocariasis is reported in Japan, Correa, France, Brazil, and the USA, while neuro-toxocariasis is dominant in Europe, Asia, and the Americas, and visceral larva migrans reports are coming from Spain, India, Argentina, and Brazil. In developed countries, humans are most commonly infected with Toxocara spp. Eggs contaminated soil, food, and water. Dogs and cats are the main source of contamination, especially in communities where these animals have free access to public parks and playgrounds. In some countries such as the United Kingdom foxes became a primary contaminant of the environment. Contamination of soil of public parks in most countries varies within a range of 17.4–60.3% according to reports from Brazil, 14.4–20.6% in the USA, 13.0–87.1% in Europe, 30.3–54.5% in Africa, and 6.6–63.3% in Asia [19]. Also, humans can be infected with embryonated eggs attached to the hair of dogs and cats. In accordance with the wide para-enteritis host range, some human cases are associated with the consumption of undercooked beef, lamb, and chicken. Besides Toxocara spp., other geo-helminths represent a significant problem in tropic and subtropic regions. Most important are *Ascaris* spp., *Ancylostoma* spp., *Uncinaria stenocephala*, *Trichuris* spp., and *Strongyloides stercoralis*. According to the WHO reports almost 1.5 billion people are exposed to these parasites. Infection occurs most commonly by ingestion of eggs, by feco-oral route, or penetration of larvae from the soil through host skin [20]. Geo-helminths in humans causes a range of different, non-specific symptoms, hypersensitivity, small intestine obstruction, volvulus or intussusception, cholecystitis, and pancreatitis. Anemia can occur due to mucosal bleeding from the upper gastrointestinal system. Patients with severe disease demonstrate eosinophilic pneumonia, urticaria, cough, dyspnea, hemoptysis, pleuritis, pleural exudate, hepatic abscesses, diarrhea, dermatitis, asthenia, abdominal pain, tachycardia, tachypnea, edema, hematochezia, and occasionally melena. Diagnosis is by parasitological examination and identification of eggs or adults in feces, sputum, bronchoscopy, endoscopy, basic blood analysis, serological tests, and imaging techniques. Treatment includes the administration of antibiotics and anthelmintics (albendazole, mebendazole, ivermectin). With small intestine obstruction, volvulus, or intussusception, surgical laparotomy is indicated.

Dirofilariosis is a mosquito-borne zoonotic disease caused by the nematode of the genus *Dirofilaria*. Several species of this genus may cause human infection; *D. repens*, *D. immitis*, *D. tenuis*, *D. striata, D. ursi,* and others. Adult forms of *D. repens* are parasites of skin and subcutaneous tissues of animals, while *D. immitis*, known as "heartworms", is usually found in pulmonary arteries and right hearth of dogs and other carnivores. *D. tenuis* infects raccoons, *D. striata* wild felids and *D. ursi* is found in bears [21]. Animals are considered natural hosts while humans are accidental hosts. Increased occurrence of dirofilariasis is reported in Europe related to traveling in endemic areas. Human dirofilariasis is reported in 46 countries from five continents (Afrika, Amerika, Asia, Australia, and Europe). *D. repens* occurs in 39 countries from all continents but America, *D. immitis* is reported in 15 countries from all continents but Africa, *D. tenuis* is reported from USA and India, D. *hongkongensis* from China and Austria, *D. striata* from America and *D. ursi* from Japan [21]. The life cycle of Dirofilaria has five stages developing invertebrate hosts and mosquitos as vectors (dominantly *Culex* spp. and *Aedes* spp.). Mosquitoes transmit third-stage larvae. In the host body nodules are formed at different locations depending on which ocular, subcutaneous and pulmonal dirofilariasis is developed. Since symptoms are absent or non-specific diagnosis is complex. The most common signs are redness of the eye, irritation, and pain similar to allergy conjunctivitis. Diagnosis is by examination of nodules and by x-rays. Therapy consists of surgical removal of nodules from lungs and subcutis. In most cases, treatment with antiparasitic is not necessary.

Capillariasis is a globally distributed zoonotic parasitosis caused by nematode *Capillaria* spp. So far over 300 species of *Capillaria* had been identified with a wide host range, while the following species cause infections in humans; *C. philippinensis*, *C. hepatica,* and *C. aerophila*. Capillariasis is the first time described in rural areas of the Philippines and Thailand, following spread to Indonesia, Japan, Taiwan, India, and Egypt [22]. Cases reported in Europe are mostly imported through travel in endemic areas. The parasite is localized in the liver of mammal hosts, particularly rodents, while humans are accidental hosts. Final hosts—rodents represent a source of environmental contamination. They are transmitted by water or food. In the liver due to parasite migration necrotic lesions, inflammations, and tissue granulation is found. In humans, capillariasis can be intestinal, pulmonal, or hepatic. Symptoms are fever, hepatomegaly, eosinophilia, and an increase in liver enzymes. Complications of infection include lobular pneumonia, pulmonary abscesses, anemia, kidney damage, splenomegaly, and congestion. Diagnosis is made by identification of eggs from stool, liver biopsy, imaging techniques, serological tests such as ELISA, and Indirect immunofluorescence (IFA). Therapy is based on thiabendazole and albendazole.

Trypanosomiasis is caused by species of the genus *Trypanosoma*. Chagas disease (CD) or American trypanosomiasis is caused by protozoa *T. cruzi*, while *T. brucei rhodesiense* and *T. brucei gambiense* are causative agents of African sleeping sickness (African trypanosomiasis). *T. cruzi* is transmitted by insects of the sub-family Triatominiae, while *T. brucei* is transmitted by tsetse flies of the genus Glossina. Both diseases are connected with high morbidity and mortality and are difficult to control since many wild and domestic animals are natural reservoirs. During the life cycle, the parasite undergoes three stages; intracellular amastigote (proliferative form found in invertebrates), epimastigotes (proliferative form from invertebrate intestines), and extracellular trypomastigote. During feeding, hematophagy insects introduce trypomastigote which transforms into epimastigotes [23]. The CD is one of the leading public health issues in most South American countries. Due to continuous migrations of people from endemic areas disease is more and more frequently reported in non-endemic areas like North America, Europe, Australia, and Japan. Here transmission occurs through blood transfusion, organ transplantation, or vertical transmission from mother to child. The disease affects about 6–8 million people worldwide, causing 50.000 deaths, while 65–100 million people live in endemic areas. *T. brucei* is an extracellular parasite found in the blood, lymph, lymphatic nods, liquor, and interstitial fluid of the host. The acute form is often fatal to a host, however, if the patient survives, the disease becomes chronic followed by migration of the parasite to cerebrospinal fluid. The patient succumbs to septicemia or meningitis. *T. cruzi* invades macrophages, fibroblast, and epithelial cells. The acute stage of infection is accompanied by high parasitemia with no symptoms or showing as fever, anorexia, and tachycardia. Diagnosis in the acute stage is based on the detection of the parasite in blood or by PCR. In the chronic stage, serological tests are used. Therapeutics (nifurtimox, benznidazole) are efficient in the acute stage of *T. cruzi* infection. For treatment of *T. brucei* infection in acute form pentamidine (*T. b. gambiense*) and suramin (*T. b. rhodesiense*) are used, while for chronic stage melarsoprol and eflornithine.

Leishmaniasis is one of the most important protozoan diseases. Causative agents are of the genus *Leishmania*, within which zoonotic are *L. infantum*, *L. donovani*, *L. peruviana*, *L. braziliensis*, *L. mexicana*, *L. major*, and others. This is a vector-borne disease transmitted by sandflies, insects of the genus *Phlebotomus* and *Lutzomyia*. Most of the species cause disease in many mammals which represent the reservoir of the parasite (rodents, dogs, cats, wolfs, and primates) [24]. Dogs are the main reservoirs in urban areas, while foxes, jacals, and wolfs are important salivatic hosts. Leishmania has a heterosexual life cycle, including two morphologically different forms; amastigote found in macrophages of domesticated mammals and promastigote found in intestines of vectors. In humans, the infection starts when female Phlebotomus inoculates promastigote through the skin. The macrophages then intake promastigote by phagocytosis where the parasite transforms into a non-flageal form—amastigote. This form is further reproduced by binary fission within macrophages. Diseases in endemic in a large number of countries mainly in South and Central America, Africa, Asia, and Mediterranean countries. Annually 1.5 million cases of cutaneous leishmaniasis are confirmed and about 500.000 cases of visceral leishmaniasis alongside 30.000 fatalities [25]. Risk factors for leishmaniasis are related to urbanization and climate changes. An increase in the average temperatures delays the reproduction season of the vector species. Hence endemic areas for zoonotic leishmaniasis had spread to northern Italy, Germany, the United Kingdom, Hungary, and France. There are two clinical manifestations of leishmaniasis in humans. Visceral leishmaniasis in humans and dogs is caused by *L. donovani* and *L. infantum*. The other species most commonly cause cutaneous or mucocutaneous disease accompanied by papulose, muco-papulose, and nodular exanthema. The visceral form is accompanied by fever, hepatosplenomegaly, pancytopenia, weakness, and weight loss. If not treated, severe cases of visceral leishmaniasis are usually fatal, due to direct effects of the disease or due to secondary complications (bacterial infection and hemorrhage). Diagnosis is made based on clinical manifestation, parasitological, serological, and molecular tests. Therapy must be adjusted to individual cases and the most commonly includes amphotericin, pentamidine, pentavalent antimonial, ketoconazole, itraconazole, fluconazole, and miltefosine.

Giardiasis is a disease caused by *Giardia duodenalis* (formerly called *G. lamblia* or G. *intestinalis*), with at least eight genotypes (A-H) confirmed in humans and other mammals. Species of the genus *Giardia* are found in other hosts; *G. agilis* in amphibia, *G. ardeae* and *G. psittaci* in birds, *G. microti* and *G. muris* in rodents [26]. Giardiasis is globally distributed, yielding over 280 million cases caused dominantly by genotypes A and B [26]. Epidemics and increases in prevalence are related to exposure to contaminated food and water, public pools, and daycare establishments. The disease is important from a veterinary perspective since it causes serious symptoms in animals as well as death, while diseased animals are a source of infection for humans. The life cycle of *Giardia* includes two phases; trophozoite (replicating stage) and cyst (infectious stage). Infection can occur directly by ingestion of cysts or by the feco-oral route. The following infection in the duodenum, cyst transforms to trophozoite, which reproduces by binary division, forming the cysts then excreted by feces. Cysts are very viable and can maintain infectivity in the environment for weeks and months. The disease can be asymptomatic or in acute form followed by dehydration, abdominal pain, nausea, vomiting, and weight loss. In the chronic form, the disease can manifest as the syndrome of irritable colon and chronic fatigue. Laboratory diagnosis of *Giardia* spp. Is mainly based on the detection of cysts or trophozoite in fecal samples by serological and molecular methods. Treatment is adjusted to anamnesis and clinical findings and includes metronidazole, tinidazole, nitazoxanide, paromomycin, quinacrine, and furazolidone.

Malaria is a disease caused by the parasites of the genus *Plasmodium*. Species found in humans are *P. malariae*, *P. falciparum*, *P. vivax*, *P. ovale,* and *P. knowlesi*. The disease is transmitted by mosquitoes of the genus *Anopheles* which transmit disease to humans and other vertebrates [27]. Malaria is still one of the most severe diseases affecting hundreds of million people worldwide causing over 400.000 deaths annually. *P. vivax*, in most cases considered the cause of re-emergent malaria occurrence, is an ancient and common zoonosis originating from apes. The occurrence of other zoonotic malaria agents (*P. knowlesi*, *P. cynomolgi,* and *P. simium*) additionally accentuates the severity of this disease. Malaria is the most common in Africa and some Asian countries. Species found in America and Europe are *P. vivax* and *P. malariae*, while in Africa dominant species is *P. falciparum*. The life cycle is very complex and evolves in two stages; sexual in mosquitoes and asexual in vertebrates including humans [27]. Clinical symptoms of malaria; fever, nausea, and weakness are related to every cycle of merozoite exiting and leaving erythrocytes. Diagnostic tests for malaria include microscopic analysis of blood smears (golden standard), PCR, IFA, and ELISA. Treatment of malaria is based on anti-malaria drugs; chloroquine phosphates, with increasing reports of resistance to this drug from around the world. Other drugs are used in addition such as primaquine, and quinine sulfate alongside doxycycline and mefloquine.

Toxoplasmosis is an important disease in animals and humans globally, especially due to resulting in stillbirths and miscarriages in humans [28]. The causative agent, *Toxoplasma gondii* can be found in many species of animals and humans. More than a billion people in the world are infected by *T. gondii*, with very high seroprevalence in some countries (Brazil, 77.5%; St. Thomas and Principe, 75.2%; Iran, 63.9%; Columbia, 63.5%; and Cuba, 61.8%). Only in the USA, the annual cumulative incidence is 9.832 new cases; out of which 2.169 are ocular form and 1.399 cerebral forms of toxoplasmosis as the most common form of the disease [28]. Humans and most warm-blooded animals and intermediate hosts, while domestic and other cats are final hosts. In the final host's intestines, parasites reproduce sexually, resulting in forming of the oocyst, which matures by sporulation to an infectious form. People get infected by consumption of raw or undercooked meat (mainly lamb and pork) containing bradyzoites or ingestion of the sporulated oocysts found on vegetables, water, in cat feces, transmission from mother to a child, or by organ transplantation. In most patients, primary infection or mild form when parasites are found in different organs, mainly the heart and skeletal muscles, brain, and retina. Alongside three standard forms of toxoplasmosis (ocular, congenital, and cerebral), a latent infection occurs characterized by behavioral changes and neurologic symptoms. Diagnosis is made by imagining techniques, histopathology, and serological test. Dormant parasites in tissues are the main obstacle to successful treatment since no drug available can reach the parasites encapsulated in cysts. Currently available drugs are efficient for acute and reactivated infections caused by tachyzoites. If treatment is not timely, a fatal outcome is inevitable in immunocompromised individuals. Therapy includes derivates of pyrimethamine in combination with sulfadiazine or clindamycin.

Cryptosporidiosis is caused by the species of the genus *Cryptosporidium* resulting in intestinal infections in a large number of vertebrates including humans, wildlife, reptiles, birds, amphibian, and fish [25]. Species the most commonly found in humans are *C. parvum* and *C. hominis,* causing over 90% of cases of cryptosporidiosis, and also *C. meleagridis* along with other parasite species. *C. parvum* has a range of hosts that includes over one hundred mammal species demonstrating the excellent adaptation of the parasite [29]. *Cryptosporidium* can be found in water, food, and surfaces contaminated with feces. The infection comes with ingestion of contaminated water, food, or by direct contact (community and hospital infections). The *Cryptosporidium* due to its morphological features can persist for longer periods outside the host and is very resistant to many desificants. Development of the *C. parvum* starts with sporulated oocytes, which after ingestion begin asexual (merogonial) and sexual (gametogonia) reproduction in small intestines. The significance of this infection reflects in high incidence especially in children, immunocompromised parsons (AIDS patients) with the highest case fatality rate in younger individuals. The most common symptom is diarrhea followed by dehydration, nausea, vomiting, increased temperature, and weight loss [29]. All domestic and wild animals, as well as humans, can serve as potential reservoirs resulting in contamination of food and water, while feco-oral transmission is also possible. The disease is globally distributed and, in the USA, Canada, Australia, and Europe it is considered one of the most common water borne pathogens. Diagnosis is established by examination of dyed fecal smears, serological tests, and PCR. The USA Food and Drug Administration approved nitazoxanide for human therapy.

Babesiosis is a tick-borne disease caused by the parasites of the genus *Babesia*. Over 100 species of *Babesia* are described, most causing high morbidity in animals, while only some are competent human pathogens. Disease transmission occurs by bite of an infected tick, blood transfusion, or via the placenta. Babesiosis is confirmed on all continents with *B. microti* (rodents) found in North America, *B. divergens* (cattle) most commonly found in Europe, and some infections by *B. duncani* and *B. venatorum* [30]. The occurrence of babesiosis is related to tick distribution and competent vector species of ticks are *Ixodes scapularis, I. ricinus,* and *I. persulcatus*. *Babesia* can be found also in tick species *Dermacentor reticulatus*, *D. marginatus*, *D. silvarum*, *Haemaphysalis longicornis*, *H. punctata*, *H. concinna*, *H. leporispalustris*, *H. japonica*, *H. sulcata*, *Hyalomma marginatum*, *Amblyomma variegatum*, *Argas (Carios) vespertilionis*, *Rhipicephalus simus*, *R. turanicus*, *R. bursa*, *R. microplus,* and *R. sanguineus*. Global annual prevalence is 12.45%; largest in North America (27.81%), Europe (9.88%), Asia (9.30%) and Africa (8.55%) [30]. Human infection is mostly asymptomatic, sometimes with fever, headache, lethargy, loss of appetite, nausea, and dyspnea. Older and immunocompromised individuals are at greater risk of developing more severe symptoms such as hepatomegaly and kidney failure. Diagnosis is made by macroscopical examination of blood smears. Patients with mild disease receive therapy of atovaquone and azithromycin, while in severe cases clindamycin and kinin are used. Since currently there is no vaccine available, recommendations are to avoid tick bites using repellents and appropriate clothing. Babesiosis gains more priority for control due to the risks of its spread influenced by climate changes, vector distribution, and a huge impact on public health.

Amebiasis is a disease caused by *Entamoeba hystolitica* leading to dysentery in humans. It is transmitted by contaminated food, and water and results in a high case fatality rate especially in children from poor countries [31]. In addition to humans E. *histolytica* can be found in primates, cats, dogs, and other animals such as mice and pigs serving as reservoirs. Besides *E. hystolitica* other parasitic species are recorded; *E. dispar*, *E. moshkovskii*, *E. coli*, *E. hartmanni*. *E. histolytica* is globally distributed, with the highest occurrence in tropical and sub-tropical regions of South America, Africa, and Asia, especially in rural areas with poor sanitary conditions and malnutrition. Amebiasis follows giardiasis and campylobacteriosis is the leading cause of gastrointestinal disease in humans. The life cycle of *E. histolytica* is relatively simple and has two stages; cysts and vegetative trophozoite. Mature cysts as an infectious form of the parasite are found in feces, while trophozoites invasive form are in epithelial cells of the intestine. By feco-oral route and ingestion by food and water infectious cysts of *E. histolytica* passage through the stomach, mature in the ileum into trophozoite which colonizes the large intestine and destroys epithelial cells causing inflammation and dysentery. Parasites can by portal vein reach the liver and cause extraintestinal infection followed by liver, lung, or brain abscesses [32]. Clinical symptoms vary from diarrhea to severe dysentery accompanied by abdominal pain, and watery or bloody stool. Diagnosis by symptoms is difficult, hence parasitological, serological, and molecular tests are used. The ELISA antigen test is available, while out of molecular assays conventional and multiplex PCR are used as well as Loop-mediated isothermal amplification test (LAMP). Treatment includes amebicides such as metronidazole, emetine, chloroquine, diloxanide-furoate, and some antibiotics (tetracycline, paromomycin, erythromycin).

5. Prevention and control of parasitic diseases

The constant increase in numbers of human parasitoses is being reported worldwide, while zoonotic parasites are among the most important causes of human infectious diseases, especially in undeveloped and developing countries [8]. Parasitoses make up the majority of the WHO/FAO lists of the NTDs, affecting 1000 million people in endemic areas, including 149 countries [7]. Causes for a surge of zoonotic parasitic infections in humans and the emergence of zoonotic parasites are various, such as overpopulation, migrations due to natural or man-made disasters, inadequate food and water supplies, encroachment leading to human interaction with new animal and/or parasite species and global warming influencing distribution and survival of parasites with resultant overflow infections [32, 33]. The consideration that parasitic diseases are exclusively associated with tropical and/or undeveloped countries with deficient hygienic and sanitary conditions in recent years has been widely challenged. The developed countries have witnessed an unprecedented increase of some parasitosis due to migrations, tourism, changing alimentary customs, and internationalization of commerce [34]. Parasitic infections are even more a threat to immunocompromised people due to genetic, iatrogenic, or infectious causes.

The surveillance of zoonotic parasites is important for common health and begins with an investigation of the presence of known and potentially zoonotic parasites in both human and animal populations and the environment. Estimating the extent of the parasites worldwide is hampered since in many countries they are not notifiable diseases, while in addition, the parasitosis can be asymptomatic or with an unspecific symptom that makes its diagnosis difficult [34]. The traditional approach to the prevention of parasitic infection in animals is based on chemoprophylaxis and treatments are commonly not scheduled, nor they are regular or specific and rely on owners' awareness and initiative. In humans particularly in endemic areas regular and mass treatment is considered the main approach for infection control [4]. However, costs associated with diagnosis and prevention in animals and animal origin food are lesser than the mass treatment and diverse consequences of parasitic infections in humans [35]. Unselective treatment with anti-parasitic drugs has also brought to the light issue of resistance. According to Moleto [36] use of the broad spectrum anthelmintics started in the early 60s had superior outcomes, but the present situation is worsening with alarming consequences arising from the development of the multidrug-resistant parasite population. Currently, other means of parasitic infection control in animals are developed such as vaccination, breeding for resistance, biological control, and grazing management [36].

Since the animals and the environment are the main sources of infection for humans, control of zoonotic parasitoses needs to be primarily addressed at these levels. Rapid, simple, and available diagnostic methods are available for the detection of parasites in both companion and food animals and environmental samples, thus enabling early detection and specific treatment. Alongside investigations of parasitic infection in hosts, vectors require investigation and control (i.e., ticks, mosquitoes, sand flies, etc.). The trends toward an increase in vector populations are, in part, due to landscape fragmentation and an increase in the abundance of hosts. This, along with warming temperatures, has enabled the gaining vector competency, development, and survival of many vector species not as earlier limited by the season (temperatures and precipitation), altitude, and geographical distribution [37]. In the past dominant source of parasite infection in humans was infested animal origin food, which still is important but the majority of human infection nowadays is linked to companion animals and outdoor activities (contaminated environment and vectors).

Further down the food chain control of food-borne parasitoses in animal origin food needs to be part of sanitary and quality control in food processing establishments (i.e., slaughterhouses) [35]. In addition to regulated meat inspection, other methods have become available such as commercial serologic detection kits (for screening antibodies in milk) and near-infrared hyperspectral imaging (for animal carcasses inspection) [35, 38]. Besides direct consequences on human health through parasite-infested food, parasitic diseases such as gastrointestinal parasitoses in food animals are the single most important cause of production losses [36]. Parasite infections are shown to significantly affect milk yield, lower milk protein content, impair fertility, and contribute to a more frequent onset of metabolic disorders in animals as well as cause condemnation of affected organs (i.e., liver) [38]. Considering traditionally low animal productivity in undeveloped and developing countries, simultaneously struggling with many animals health issues, further decrease in the availability of animal protein due to parasitism is a serious threat to food security, nutrition-related deficiency, and both the health and economic wellbeing of humans (**Figure 2**). Also, in developed countries, changes in production due to animal welfare

Parasitic diseases in food animals		
Production losses		Increased cost and negative consequences
Economic - reduced production - vaccination - chemoprophylaxix - biosecurity - restriction of movement and trade	Social - animal welfare - zoonotic parasitic diseases - reduced food availability - malnutrition	Environmental - greenhouse gases - ecotoxicity - environmental residues of antibiotics and aanhelmintics - inefficient land and water use

Figure 2.
Impact of parasite infection in food animals [39].

perspectives (i.e., pasture access) and an increase in organic farming led to altered patterns of parasite prevalence in farmed animals. For example, an increase in *F. hepatica* prevalence and/or an increase in the geographical spread of this parasite alongside recognition of its zoonotic potential has been observed in some European countries during recent years [38].

Control of parasitic infections is difficult for various reasons. First, many of these parasitoses are zoonosis, which requires collaboration between the human and animal health sector. It was long recognized that many emerging zoonoses arise from complex, diverse, and constantly evolving factors related to the environment, people, and animals. Zoonotic parasitoses with emergence and adaptability, wide host range, and various means of transmission all highly influenced by the environment need One Health approaches in both investigations, health regulations, prevention, and control measures [40]. On the other hand, the socio-economic conditions of developing countries make it difficult to apply measures to prevent or combat these diseases. Research on vaccines is yet expected to produce applicable results, while sophisticated molecular diagnostics on a routine basis are not even done in developed countries.

6. Conclusion and recommendations

Parasitoses of humans and animals contribute significantly to a global burden of infectious diseases, public health, animal health, and production, especially considering current trends of disease emergence and re-emergence and the high and increasing dominance of zoonotic pathogens. Research shows that exposure and increased risk of zoonotic pathogens are influenced by global environmental, social, and economic trends mainly man-made. Understanding, predicting, addressing, and preventing diseases with fast-evolving virulence, host range, pathogenesis and epidemiology require multidisciplinary approaches and reactions. Genesis as well as consequences of novel and re-emerging pathogens is complex, hence it needs to be addressed in its entirety to be proactive. Researchers, international bodies, governments, and the entire global community are called to adopt and adapt in their efforts to combat common health and wellbeing threats either current or those inevitably looming over the horizon.

Author details

Jasmin Omeragic, Sabina Seric-Haracic* and Naida Kapo
Veterinary Faculty, University of Sarajevo, Sarajevo, Bosnia and Herzegovina

*Address all correspondence to: sabina.seric-haracic@vfs.unsa.ba

References

[1] Lindgren E, Talleklint L, Polfeldt T. Impact of climatic change on the northern latitude limit and population density of the disease-transmitting European tick Ixodes ricinus. Environmental Health Perspectives. 2000;**108**:119-123. DOI: 10.1289/ehp.00108119

[2] Ndimubanzi PC, Carabin H, Budke CM, Nguyen H, Qian YJ, Rainwater E, et al. A systematic review of the frequency of neurocysticercosis with a focus on people with epilepsy. PLoS Neglected Tropical Diseases. 2010;**4**:870. DOI: 10.1371/journal.pntd.0000870

[3] White RJ, Razgour O. Emerging zoonotic diseases originating in mammals: A systematic review of effects of anthropogenic land-use change. Mammal Review. 2020;**50**(4):336-352. DOI: 10.1111/mam.12201

[4] Babu S, Nutman TB. Immune responses to helminth infection. In: Rich RR, Fleisher TA, Shearer WT, Schroeder HW, Frew AJ, Weyand CM, editors. Clinical Immunology. 5th ed. London: Elsevier; 2019. pp. 437-447.e1. DOI: 10.1016/B978-0-7020-6896-6.00031-4

[5] Montoya JG, Liesenfeld O. Toxoplasmosis. The Lancet. 2004;**363**:1965-1976. DOI: 10.1016/S0140-6736(04)16412-X

[6] Efstratiou A, Ongerth JE, Karanis P. Waterborne transmission of protozoan parasites: Review of worldwide outbreaks—An update 2011-2016. Water Research. 2017;**114**:14-22. DOI: 10.1016/j.watres.2017.01.036

[7] World Health Organization & Food and Agriculture Organization of the United Nations. Multicriteria-based ranking for risk management of food-borne parasites. In: Report of a Joint FAO/WHO Expert Meeting; 3-7 September 2012; Italy. Rome: FAO, World Health Organization; 2014. p. 302

[8] Mascarini-Serra L. Prevention of soil-transmitted helminth infection. Journal of Global Infectious Diseases. 2011;**3**:175-182. DOI: 10.4103/0974-777X.81696

[9] Baumann S, Shi R, Liu W, Bao H, Schmidberger J, Kratzer W, et al. Interdisciplinary Echinococcosis Working Group Ulm. Worldwide literature on the epidemiology of human alveolar echinococcosis: A systematic review of research published in the twenty-first century. Infection. 2019;**47**:703-727. DOI: 10.1007/s15010-019-01325-2

[10] Maleki B, Dalimi A, Majidiani H, Badri M, Gorgipour M, Khorshidi A. Parasitic infections of wild boars (*Sus scrofa*) in Iran: A literature review. Infectious Disorders-Drug Targets (Formerly Current Drug Targets-Infectious Disorders). 2020;**20**:585-597. DOI: 10.2174/187152651966619071612182

[11] Caravedo MA, Cabada MM. Human fascioliasis: Current epidemiological status and strategies for diagnosis, treatment, and control. Research and Reports in Tropical Medicine. 2020;**11**:149-158. DOI: 10.2147/RRTM.S237461

[12] Alba A, Vazquez AA, Hurtrez-Boussès S. Towards the comprehension of fasciolosis (re-) emergence: An integrative overview. Parasitology. 2021;**148**:385-407. DOI: 10.1017/S0031182020002255

[13] McManus DP, Dunne DW, Sacko M, Utzinger J, Vennervald BJ, Zhou XN.

Schistosomiasis. Nature Reviews Disease Primers. 2018;**4**:13. DOI: 10.1038/s41572-018-0013-8

[14] Saijuntha W, Sithithaworn P, Petney TN, Andrews RH. Foodborne zoonotic parasites of the family Opisthorchiidae. Research in Veterinary Science. 2021;**135**:404-411. DOI: 10.1016/j.rvsc.2020.10.024

[15] Woolsey ID, Miller AL. Echinococcus granulosus sensu lato and Echinococcus multilocularis: A review. Research Veterinary Science. 2021;**135**:517-522. DOI: DOPI: 10.1016/j.rvsc.2020.11.010

[16] Singh RP, Roy BC, Debnath AK, Nahar SF, Talukder MH. Hymenolepiasis in rats (*Rattus norvegicus*) with its zoonotic potential in Mymensingh District of Bangladesh. Research in Agriculture Livestock and Fisheries. 2020;7:255-259. DOI: 10.3329/ralf.v7i2.48865

[17] Symeonidou I, Arsenopoulos K, Tzilves D, Soba B, Gabriël S, Papadopoulos E. Human taeniasis/cysticercosis: A potentially emerging parasitic disease in Europe. Annals of Gastroenterology. 2018;**31**:406-412. DOI: 10.20524/aog.2018.0260

[18] Murrell KD, Pozio E. Trichinellosis: The zoonosis that won't go quietly. International Journal for Parasitology. 2000;**30**:1339-1349. DOI: 10.1016/s0020-7519(00)00132-6

[19] Chen J, Liu Q, Liu GH, Zheng WB, Hong SJ, Sugiyama H, et al. Toxocariasis: A silent threat with a progressive public health impact. Infectious Disease Poverty. 2018;7:59. DOI: 10.1186/s40249-018-0437-0

[20] Jourdan PM, Lamberton PHL, Fenwick A, Addiss DG. Soil-transmitted helminth infections. Lancet. 2018;**391**:252-265. DOI: 10.1016/S0140-6736(17)31930-X

[21] Pupić-Bakrač A, Pupić-Bakrač J, Beck A, Jurković D, Polkinghorne A, Beck R. Regarding 'Human dirofilariasis in the 21st century: A scoping review of clinical cases reported in the literature. Transboundary and Emerging Diseases. 2021:1-16. DOI: 10.1111/tbed.14431

[22] Dubey A, Bagchi A, Sharma D, Dey A, Nandy K, Sharma R. Hepatic Capillariasis-drug targets. Infectious Disorders—Drug Targets. 2018;**18**:3-10. DOI: 10.2174/1871526517666170427124254

[23] Kirchhoff LV, Bacchi CJ, Machado FS, Weiss HD, Huang H, Mukherjee S, et al. Trypanosomes. In: Encyclopedia of Microbiology. Amsterdam, Netherlands: Elsevier Inc; 2009. pp. 744-757. DOI: 10.1016/B978-012373944-5.00211-X

[24] Mohebali M, Moradi-Asl E, Rassi Y. Geographic distribution and spatial analysis of *Leishmania infantum* infection in domestic and wild animal reservoir hosts of zoonotic visceral leishmaniasis in Iran: A systematic review. Journal of Vector-Borne Diseases. 2018;**55**:173-183. DOI: 10.4103/0972-9062.249125

[25] Plutzer J, Lassen B, Jokelainen P, Djurković-Djaković O, Kucsera I, Dorbek-Kolin E, et al. Review of *Cryptosporidium* and *Giardia* in the eastern part of Europe 2016. Euro Surveillance. 2018;**23**:16-00825. DOI: 10.2807/1560-7917.ES.2018.23.4.16-00825

[26] Wang Y, Gonzalez-Moreno O, Roellig MD, Oliver L, Huguet J, Guo Y, et al. Epidemiological distribution of genotypes of *Giardia duodenalis* in humans in Spain. Parasites & Vectors. 2019;**12**:432. DOI: 10.1186/s13071-019-3692-4

[27] Hang JW, Tukijan F, Lee EQ, Abdeen SR, Aniweh Y, Malleret B. Zoonotic malaria: Non-Laverania plasmodium biology and invasion mechanisms. Pathogens. 2021;**10**:889. DOI: 10.3390/pathogens10070889

[28] Elsheikha HM, Marra CM, Zhu XQ. Epidemiology, pathophysiology, diagnosis, and management of cerebral toxoplasmosis. Clinical Microbiology Reviews. 2020;**34**:e00115-e00119. DOI: 10.1128/CMR.00115-19

[29] Putignani L, Menichella D. Global distribution, public health and clinical impact of the protozoan pathogen cryptosporidium. Interdisciplinary Perspectives on Infectious Diseases. 2010;**753512**. DOI: 10.1155/2010/753512

[30] Karshima SN, Karshima MN, Ahmed MI. Animal reservoirs of zoonotic Babesia species: A global systematic review and meta-analysis of their prevalence, distribution and species diversity. Veterinary Parasitology. 2021;**298**:109539. DOI: 10.1016/j.vetpar.2021.109539

[31] Junaidi J, Cahyaningsih U, Purnawarman T, Latif H, Sudarnika E, Hayati Z, et al. Entamoeba histolytica neglected tropical diseases (NTDs) agents that infect humans and some other mammals: A review. E3S Web of Conferences. 2020;**151**:01019. DOI: 10.1051/e3sconf/20201510101

[32] Chomel BB. Control and prevention of emerging parasitic zoonoses. International Journal of Parasitology. 2008;**38**:1211-1217. DOI: 10.1016/j.ijpara.2008.05.001

[33] Hoberg EP, Polley L, Jenkins EJ, Kutz SJ, Veitch AM, Elkin BT. Integrated approaches and empirical models for investigation of parasitic diseases in northern wildlife. Emerging Infectious Diseases. 2008;**14**:10-17. DOI: 10.3201/eid1401.071119

[34] Garrido-Cardenas JA, Mesa-Valle C, Manzano-Agugliaro F. Human parasitology worldwide research. Parasitology. 2018;**145**:699-712. DOI: 10.1017/S0031182017001718

[35] Zolfaghari Emameh R, Purmonen S, Sukura A, Parkkila S. Surveillance and diagnosis of zoonotic foodborne parasites. Food Science & Nutrition. 2018;**6**:3-17. DOI: 10.1002/fsn3.530

[36] Molento MB. Parasite control in the age of drug resistance and changing agricultural practices. Veterinary Parasitology. 2009;**163**:229-234. DOI: 10.1016/j.vetpar.2009.06.007

[37] Omeragić J, Šerić-Haračić S, Soldo DK, Kapo N, Fejzić N, Škapur V, et al. Distribution of ticks in Bosnia and Herzegovina. Ticks and tick-Borne Diseases. 2022;**13**:101870. DOI: 10.1016/j.ttbdis.2021.101870

[38] Springer A, Jordan D, Kirse A, Schneider B, Campe A, Knubben-Schweizer G, et al. Seroprevalence of major pasture-borne parasitoses (gastrointestinal nematodes, liver flukes, and lungworms) in German dairy cattle herds, association with management factors and impact on production parameters. Animals. 2021;**11**:2078. DOI: 10.3390/ani11072078

[39] Rushton J, Bruce M. Using a one health approach to assess the impact of parasitic disease in livestock: How does it add value? Parasitology. 2017;**144**:15-25. DOI: 10.1017/S0031182016000196

[40] Schurer JM, Mosites E, Li C, Meschke S, Rabinowitz P. Community-based surveillance of zoonotic parasites in a 'one health' world: A systematic review. One Health. 2016;**2**:166-174. DOI: 10.1016/j.onehlt.2016.11.002

Chapter 6

The Prevalence and Risk Factors Associated with Tungiasis Infestations in Uganda: Implications for Vector Borne and Neglected Tropical Disease Control

Moses Adriko

Abstract

Tungiasis is a neglected parasitic inflammatory tropical skin disease affecting the world's poorest people caused by a female flea called *Tunga penetrans*. It is potentially endemic in 88 countries worldwide, with an estimated community prevalence of 60%. The national prevalence is estimated at 50% with recent epidemics re-emergence dimensions in Uganda. The disease burden continues to escalate with high-school dropouts, absenteeism, and poor performance. This study was geared toward assessing the prevalence and risk factors in communities in Uganda. Overall, there is prevalence of 40.6 and 28% among households and individuals. Our findings further indicate prevalence of infection was the highest at household level compared to infected individuals observed; (Jinja; 73.3% vs. 50.0%), (Namutumba; 53.2% vs. 33.3%), (Iganga; 41.1% vs. 25.3%), (Bugiri; 24.4% vs. 27.1%), (Namayingo; 20.5% vs. 12.6%) and (Mayuge; 13.6% vs. 6.2%). Physical examinations revealed the most affected body parts were the toes (6.5%), sole (1.2%), and the heel (0.8%). The common method of prevention and treatment used is self-removal (49.4%), removal by a family member (32.7%), support from medical personnel (14.4%), and use of ointment (1.9%). The findings have implications for the prevention and control of Tungiasis as a public health concern in Uganda. This requires strengthened health education aimed at improved household sanitation and hygiene with community empowerment as a long-term measure.

Keywords: prevalence, risk factors, Tungiasis, Uganda, implications, control

1. Introduction

Tungiasis is a neglected tropical parasitic inflammatory tropical skin disease (NTD) affecting the world's poorest people [1] caused by a female flea called *Tunga penetrans* [2]. It is described as "the greatest curse that has ever afflicted Africa" [3] and is potentially endemic in 88 countries worldwide with an estimated prevalence in community based-settings 60% [4–9]. It is predominantly a health problem in the tropical areas of Latin America and Africa [10, 11]. It is more common in places with poor hygiene and is closely associated with domestic animals (mainly pigs, dogs, and cattle) [12]. Tungiasis commonly known as *emvunza* or *Nyende* in eastern Uganda has reemerged as the national prevalence in Uganda is estimated at 50% and recently reemerged to epidemic dimensions in many countries [13] including Uganda with an estimated prevalence of 50% reported [14, 15].

Tungiasis is a neglected disease of marginalized populations [16] and has been associated with a number of potential reservoirs from pigs, dogs, goats, mice, rats, and wild animals [17–20]. Studies have shown significant levels of infestations of goats in Uganda with Tungiasis as a serious health concern in domestic animals in Uganda including goats [21], pigs, and dogs [22]. Tungiasis is estimated to affect over 6,000,000 million people who are at risk and an estimated 3 million Ugandans infested with Tungiasis, 50% of whom, are confined to eastern Uganda especially the Busoga sub-region, the rest distributed in other regions of Karamoja and central sub-regions [23].

The ranging disease burden continues to escalate with high school dropouts, absenteeism, poor performance, and low esteem have continued to ruin the areas of Busoga region. There has been no study done to establish the magnitude of this problem and yet resource allocation and interventions can only be appropriately sought when such estimates are made. This study was geared towards assessing the prevalence and risk factors that will help provide the cornerstone for controlling future infections in communities in Uganda.

2. Materials and methods

2.1 Study area and design

This was a cross-sectional and multistage sampling study design that utilized semi-structured questionnaires combined with an observation-checklist to collect quantitative data from 983 individuals and 288 households from Bugiri, Iganga, Jinja, Namutumba, Namayingo, and Mayuge districts in eastern Uganda. The study sites are shown in **Figure 1**. The study was conducted in Bugiri, Iganga, Jinja, Namutumba, Namayingo and Mayuge districts (**Figure 1**). These districts were chosen due to the highest epidemiological reports by the Ministry of Health (weekly epidemiological reports). A sampling frame was established and randomization of the villages was performed to generate a proportional number of participants per District.

2.2 Survey methodology

The study utilized a census-style survey conducted across all the six districts survey. Overall a total of 983 individuals and 288 households were surveyed and interviewed over an eight-week period beginning February 2018. Before interviews began, an advocacy meeting was held with all the district officials to discuss the study and obtain district approval and support for the survey. Meetings were also held with the local council, chairpersons from the two villages, and the village health teams (VHTs). During mobilization meetings, community members were asked to provide information when the researchers arrived in their homes but were informed that they had no obligation to do so. Households were visited door-to-door; if residents were absent, teams returned to the house at least twice for follow-up. Informed consent

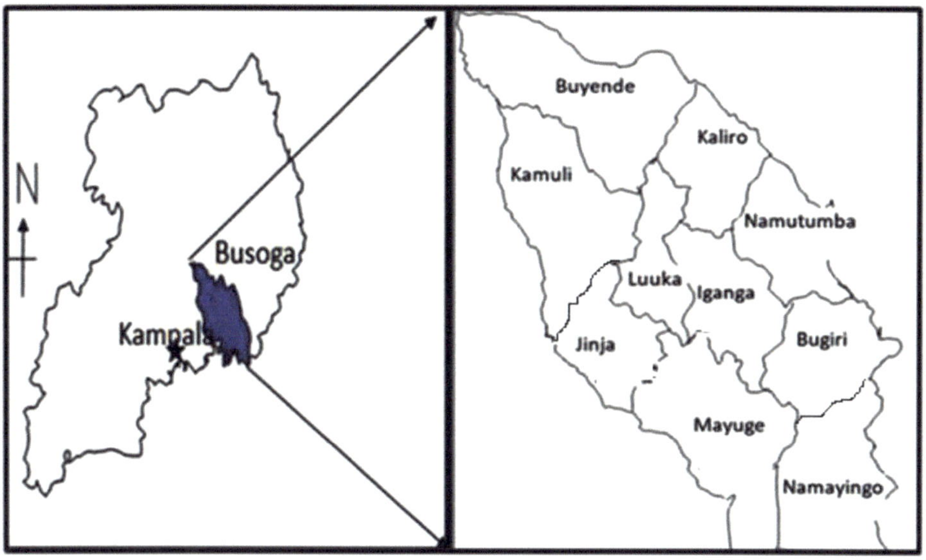

Figure 1.
Location of study area.

from the head of the household and adults present during the interview was obtained. The main interviewers were Ministry of Health Vector Control Officers or the District Health Drug Distributor and each team had a member of the Village Health Team from the respective village. There were three teams performing interviews; team members rotated between groups to ensure uniform questioning across the community.

2.3 Case definition

A short description of Tunga penetrans as an inflammatory of the skin characterized by a white patch with a black spot at the center of a swollen red lesion causing a painful itching constituted a case definition the survey team based on to determine and score observed cases. Individuals were included in the study based on the criteria that they were aged six years and above who had lived in the selected districts for a period of one year and above and excluded in the study when found of unsound mind (very sick, unconscious, mental disturbed).

2.4 Data tools and analysis

One week of training was conducted for all the research assistants involved in this study and deployed on the basis that was able to speak the native language. The data collection tools and questionnaires were pretested in one of the areas known for Tungiasis infections and corrected for errors before use in the study sites. The data collected was entered daily in the field for all the individuals into the computer and cross-checked for consistency and validity of results. A daily data review audit was performed by research to ensure compliance with the standards set.

Household and individual survey data were cleaned and checked for consistency using custom scripts in R v. 3.2.1. Chi-squared tests were used to compare categorical data using the base R function chisq.test. Multivariate logistic regressions were created with the function glm using the binomial family to evaluate two outcome variables.

2.5 Ethical clearance

The methods in the study were reviewed and approved by the Vector Control Division Research Ethic Committee (VCDREC/090) and the graduate of the Nexus International University (VUU-PGDPH-2016-037).

3. Results

3.1 Demographic characteristics of the study respondents

The demographic characteristics of the respondents are presented in **Table 1**. Overall, a total 983 respondents were interviewed. The majority of 657(66.8%) were male and only 326 (33.2%) were female. The mean age (26.13) years (standard deviation (SD) 22.56). Regarding age, the majority 500 (50.9%) were in the age bracket of 5–17 years, 187 (19%) were above 50 years of age, 120 (12.2%) were 30–39 years, 87 (8.9%) were 40–49 years of age and the least number of respondents were 18–29 years of age. concerning occupation, the majority of the respondents 376 (38.3%) were farmers, 61 (6.2%) were doing business as their occupation and a least respondents 14 (1.4%) were engaged in other activities in order to earn a living. The biggest proportion of the respondents 449 (45.7%) were Moslems, 260 (26.4%) were Catholics, 156 (15.9%) belonged to other religions and only 118 (12%) were Pentecostals.

Regarding the water source, the majority of the respondents 373 (37.9%) obtained water for household use from the rivers/lakes/streams/pond, 328 (33.3%) used piped/protected water as a source of water, 141 (14.3%) used open well water. Concerning education, the majority 526 (53.5%) had a primary level of education, 284 (28.9%) had none as the education level, 159(16.2%) had a secondary level while the least 14 (1.4%) number of respondents had obtained tertiary education. Furthermore, the majority of 557 (56.7%) were single, 225 (22.9%) were married, 161 (16.4%) were separated/divorced and only 40 (4.1%) were widow/widower. This implies that the study was mainly dominated by single respondents.

3.2 Prevalence of Tungiasis in Busoga region

The overall prevalence of Tungiasis amongst households surveyed was 40.6% (288/984) while 28% (276/984) individuals were found infected with Tungiasis during the study as shown in **Table 2**. The prevalence at the household level was much higher than at the individual level with some villages having 100% as the case with Butangula-A in Jinja district. The findings further indicate the highest prevalence of infection at the household level versus infected individuals were observed in Jinja (73.3% vs. 50.0%), followed by Namutumba (53.2% vs. 33.3%), Iganga (41.1% vs. 25.3%), Bugiri (24.4% vs. 27.1%), Namayingo (20.5% vs. 12.6%) and Mayuge (13.6% vs. 6.2%). The study findings show that the greatest age group affected by this scourge in all the districts surveyed was 5–17 years as shown in **Table 2**.

3.3 The risk factors, morbidities, and management of Tungiasis infestations in the Busoga region

The major environmental risk factors associated with Tungiasis as reported by the respondents were; poor hygiene and sanitation. Other causes reported were;

DOI: http://dx.doi.org/10.5772/intechopen.104444

Variables	Characteristics	Frequency (n = 983)	Percentage (%)
Mean age (SD) = ±26.13 (22.56)			
Age in years	5–17 yrs	500	50.9
	18–29 yrs	89	9.1
	30–39 yrs	120	12.2
	40–49 yrs	87	8.9
	>50 yrs	187	19.0
Sex	Male	657	66.8
	Female	326	33.2
Education	None	284	28.9
	Primary	526	53.5
	Secondary	159	16.2
	Tertiary	14	1.4
Marital Status	Single	557	56.7
	Married	225	22.9
	Widow/widower	40	4.1
	Separated/divorced	161	16.4
Occupation	Farmer	376	38.3
	Business	61	6.2
	Others	14	1.4
Religion	Catholic	260	26.4
	Pentecostal	118	12.0
	Moslem	449	45.7
	Others	156	15.9
Source of water	Borehole	141	14.3
	Open well	141	14.3
	Piped/protected water	328	33.3
	River/lake/stream/pond	373	37.9

Location of Study area 15.
Tungiasis infestations of the toes, finger-nails and buttocks 17.

Table 1.
Demographic characteristics of the study population.

dirtiness, uncommented house, disposal of household wastes, and people sleeping in houses with bare soils. The study findings revealed that 344 (35.0%) agreed that poor hygiene is the most commonest cause of Tungiasis since some just dispose of household wastes outside their compounds. About 6.9% of the respondents reported sharing a residential house with domestic animals while 93.1% reported having a separate shelter for domestic animals. The type of floor material for suspected cases

District	Age (years)	Frequency (%) n = 983	Chi-value	*P*-Values
Bugiri	5–17 yrs	94 (71.8%)		
	18–29 yrs	15 (11.5%)		
	30–39 yrs	6 (4.5%)	23.934	0.004
	40–49 yrs	4 (3.1%)		
	>50 yrs	12 (9.2%)		
Mayuge	5–17 yrs	88 (69.8%)		
	18–29 yrs	0 (0%)		
	30–39 yrs	9 (7.1%)	37.982	0.001
	40–49 yrs	4 (3.2%)		
	>50 yrs	25 (19.8%)		
Namayingo	5–17 yrs	87 (61.3%)		
	18–29 yrs	0 (0%)		
	30–39 yrs	14 (9.9%)	39.066	0.001
	40–49 yrs	4 (2.8%)		
	>50 yrs	36 (25.4%)		
Jinja	5–17 yrs	93 (52.8%)		
	18–29 yrs	7 (4.0%)		
	30–39 yrs	20 (11.4%)	40.983	0.001
	40–49 yrs	12 (6.8%)		
	>50 yrs	44 (25%)		
Iganga	5–17 yrs	65 (34.8%)		
	18–29 yrs	27 (14.4%)		
	30–39 yrs	27 (14.4%)	46.256	0.001
	40–49 yrs	34 (18.2%)		
	>50 yrs	34 (18.2%)		
Namutumba	5–17 yrs	74 (33.5%)		
	18–29 yrs	40 (18.1%)		
	30–39 yrs	40 (18.1%)	48.715	0.001
	40–49 yrs	30 (13.6%)		
	>50 yrs	36 (16.3%)		

Table 2.
Prevalence of Tungiasis infestation in Busoga region.

of Tungiasis reported was bare soil, clay, and sand. These observations were seen in zoonotic nature in Uganda [21, 24]. Our findings also show that disposal of household wastes was significantly associated with (p = 0.002) with outside disposal contributing the greatest percentage of 52.3%. The presence of domestic animals at home was also significantly associated with Tungiasis infestations (p = 0.002). The study also noted that knowledge concerning the causes of Tungiasis infestations was equally significantly associated with Tungiasis infestations (p = 0.002) with poor hygiene the biggest contributor accounting for 35%. Similar observations were reported by studies on the knowledge among animal keepers [25] as shown in **Table 3**.

Table 3 presents the commonest methods of prevention and treatment used by the infected individuals; self-removal accounted for 49.4%), removal by a family member

Variables	Indicators	Frequency & % (n = 983)	Chi- value	*P*-value
Floor material	Bare soil	327 (33.3%)		
	Cow dung	141 (14.3%)		
	Concrete	141 (14.3%)	14.62	0.019
	Clay	187 (19%)		
	Sand	187 (19%)		
Latrine at home	Yes	842 (85.7%)		
	No	141 (14.3%)	9.84	0.043
Disposal household wastes	Dispose outside compound	514 (52.3%)		
	Disposed in compound	141 (14.3%)	3.66	0.002
	Burnt	141 (14.3%)		
	Pit	187 (19.0%)		
Share house with animals	Yes	68 (6.9%)		
	No	915 (93.1%)		
Animals at home	Hens	89 (9.1%)		
	Goats	89 (9.1%)		
	Cows	89 (9.1%)		
	Dogs	89 (9.1%)	23.33	0.001
	Ducks	89 (9.1%)		
	Pigs	89 (9.1%)		
	Cats	89 (9.1%)		
	Pigeons	89 (9.1%)		
	Sheep	89 (9.1%)		
	None	182 (18.5%)		
Causes of Tungiasis	Poor hygiene	344 (35.0%)		
	Sleeping on the floor	86 (8.7%)		
	Too much sunshine	85 (8.6%)	24.75	0.001
	Doesn't know	85 (8.6%)		
	Un-cemented house	87 (8.9%)		
	Dirtiness	296 (30.1%)		
Localization of infections	Toes	82 (8.3%)		
	Sole	25 (2.5%)		
	Heel	25 (2.5%)		
	Dorsal area	25 (2.5%)	32.982	0.001
	Fingers	25 (2.5%)		
	Hands	42 (4.3%)		
	Forearm	42 (4.3%)		

Variables	Indicators	Frequency & % (n = 983)	Chi- value	*P*-value
Method of treatment used	Doesn't know	294 (29.9%)		
	Health workers	148 (15.1%)	32.243	0.003
	Relatives	196 (19.9%)		
	Self-removal	345 (35.1%)		

Table 3.
Risk factors and management of Tungiasis infestation in Busoga in region.

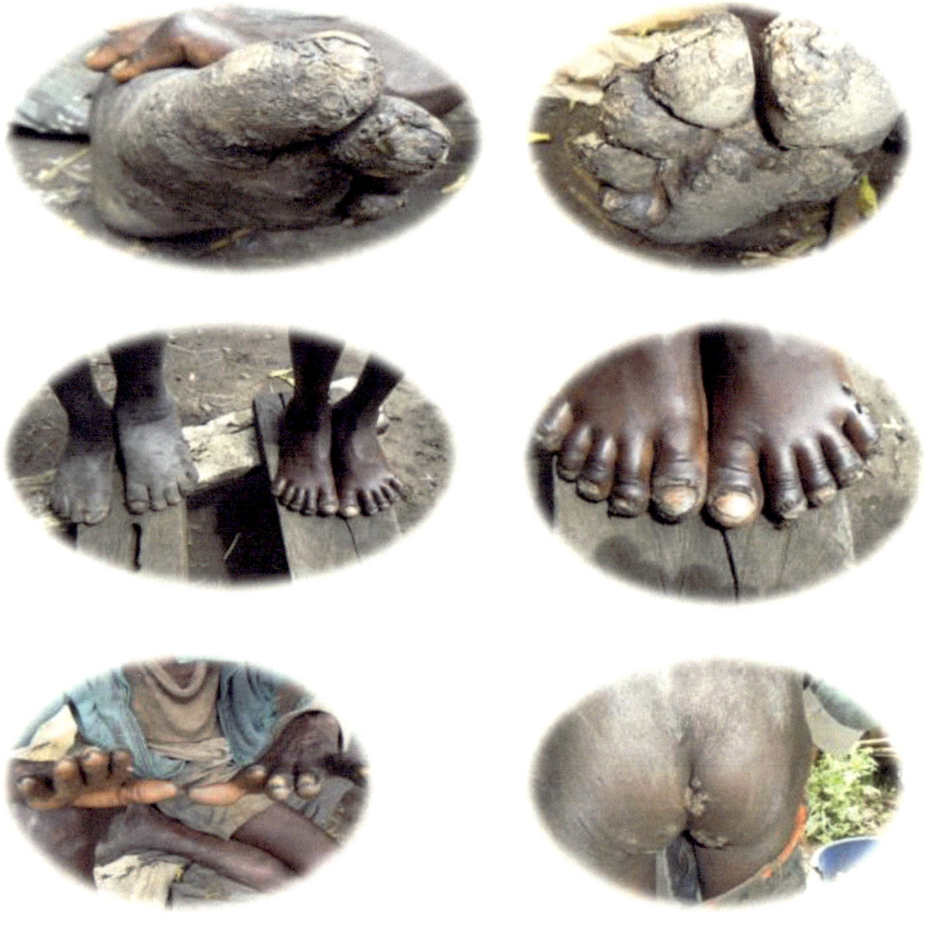

Figure 2.
Tungiasis infestations of the toe, finger-nails and buttocks.

(32.7%), support from medical personnel (14.4%), and use of ointment (1.9%). As concerns the methods of treatment for infected individuals, a bigger percentage acknowledged self-removal, 35.1%, by health workers, 15.1%, removal by relatives 19.9% and 29.9% had no idea of any interventions.

Physical examination of the respondents showed 27% (266/983) which was significantly associated with Tungiasis infections (p = 0.001) as shown in **Table 3**. The highest cumulative number of Tungiasis infections recorded was 8.35% on the toes, 2.5% on the sole, 2.5% on the heel, and 2.5% on the dorsal area. Other body parts localized with infections were the fingers (2.5%), hands (4.3%), and forearm (4.3%).

The commonest body parts affected by Tungiasis infections as shown in **Figure 2** are the fingernails, toes, buttocks, and knees.

4. Discussions

The overall prevalence of Tungiasis amongst households surveyed was 40.6% (288/984) while 28% (276/984) (95%CI, 0.0001–0.0290, $p < 0.0001$) individuals were found infected with Tungiasis during the study as shown in **Table 2**. The study findings further show that females were 2.4 times more infected with Tungiasis compared to males as observed in other studies from studies by [6, 26]. The prevalence at the household level was much higher than at the individual level with some villages having 100% as the case with Butangula-A in Jinja district. The findings further indicate the highest prevalence of infection at the household level versus infected individuals were observed in Jinja (73.3% vs. 50.0%), followed by Namutumba (53.2% vs. 33.3%), Iganga (41.1% vs. 25.3%), Bugiri (24.4%vs. 27.1%), Namayingo (20.5% vs.12.6%) and Mayuge (13.6% vs. 6.2%). The results of this study indicate that Tungiasis is a major public health problem amongst households in rural communities in eastern Uganda. The present-day study areas had previously been known as a hot spot and problematic for Tungiasis infestation in humans [15, 27] and animals [21, 22, 24, 25, 28, 29]. This could have been due to repetitive infestations of the affected households. These findings were in conformity with similar studies [28, 30].

Previous studies [26, 31] have shown that the prevalence of Tungiasis amongst 5–14 years was higher during the dry season similar to the trends observed in our study as indicated in **Table 2**. The study further points out that the prevalence of Tungiasis varied across different age groups though more significantly amongst 5–17-year-olds in almost all villages surveyed. This trend has been observed in similar studies by [8, 32], mostly attributed to the poor hygiene and exposure behaviors of these youngsters. This is made worse with the limited knowledge to take good care of themselves, frequently playing in dusty environments where the parasite thrives most.

It was a common observation that the majority of those suffering from Tungiasis infections had problems with walking because they had multiple infections on the toenails, fingernails and even to the extent some buttocks of the elderly were severely affected. Similar levels of morbidities were reported in many studies both in animals [21, 22, 29] and humans [18, 32–35] and a common cause of serious secondary bacterial infections [36].

The major environmental risk factors associated with Tungiasis as reported by the respondents were; poor hygiene and sanitation. Other causes reported were; dirtiness, uncemented house, disposal of household wastes, and people sleeping in houses with bare soils. The study findings revealed that 344 (35.0%) agreed that poor hygiene is the most commonest cause of Tungiasis since some just dispose of household wastes outside their compounds. About 6.9% of the respondents reported sharing a residential house with domestic animals while 93.1% reported having a separate shelter for domestic animals. The type of floor material for suspected cases of Tungiasis reported was bare soil, clay, and sand. These observations were seen in zoonotic nature in Uganda [21, 24]. Our findings also show that disposal of household wastes was significantly associated with ($p = 0.002$) with outside disposal contributing the greatest percentage of 52.3%. The presence of domestic animals at home was also significantly associated with Tungiasis infestations ($p = 0.002$). The study also noted that knowledge concerning the causes of Tungiasis infestations was equally significantly associated with Tungiasis infestations ($p = 0.002$) with poor hygiene the biggest contributor accounting for 35%. Similar observations were reported by studies on the knowledge among animal keepers [25]. These observations were made on studies of zoonotic nature in Uganda [21, 24]. Our findings also show that 55.4% were knowledgeable about Tungiasis infection with 23.8% reporting poor hygiene, 23.9% reporting sleeping on the floor, 24.0% stating too much sunshine, and 22.0% reporting uncemented floors as the major causes of Tungiasis infestations. Similar observations were reported by studies on the knowledge among animal keepers [25]. Only 4.5% had reported using regular footwear. The majority reported bathing with soap (73.3%) as a good strategy for the prevention of infections although only 11.5% reported having good personal hygiene as one of the prevention strategies. Physical removal of *Tunga penetrans* using manipulation with safety pin/needles accounted for 14.4%.

4.1 The National elimination Policy for Uganda

In Uganda, the disease outbreak came to light in 2010 when deaths were reported in the Bugiri district. This has resulted in a series of activities that have led to the proper understanding and recognition of Tungiasis is a neglected tropical disease. The disease is endemic in the whole country, with an estimated 6 million people are at risk and at least 2.4 million infected with Tungiasis [23]. However, 50% of total cases in Uganda come from Busoga and Karamoja Subregions. This has been included as a priority disease under the NTDs by the year 2020 through mapping to assess the distribution, Capacity building on vector control treatment and rehabilitation, Advocacy and community mobilization, Personal and Environmental hygiene, and identifying partners to support the program [23]. The warm dusty weather and environment of these regions have certainly played an amenable role in breeding Tungiasis. More so, exposed dirty floors, walls, and compounds mean Tungiasis-eggs can incubate inside homes. There are many rural families who keep animals and chickens inside their houses at night as a measure of theft. This close proximity of animals enables the transmission of eggs from animals to humans to happen with much ease.

The Ministry of Health has proposed the use of Benzyl-benzoate emulsion (BBE) combined with petroleum jelly as the medication for treating and managing cases. These have been provided to health facilities for use by the affected communities. This will be incorporated and run alongside the national control program implemented through the community-based village health teams (VHTs) geared towards community involvement and ownership. The government has proposed to strengthen and enforce the current public health act on household sanitation and hygiene, which will include smearing, cleaning, and prohibiting sharing of human dwelling houses with domestic animals. Also, strengthen community social norms with community engagement.

5. Conclusions

Based on the study findings, it's noted that Tungiasis infections present a serious health hazard to communities living in Busoga where many people live and suffer quietly under poor housing conditions. This is worsened by sharing housing and accommodation with domestic animals that are reservoirs for the infection. The following lessons have been learned during the study and recommended for further studies to advance solutions as regards the need to make a sound decision as to which drug to use during the community treatment intervention for Tungiasis. We have to choose between the scientifically backed Dimethicone (BBE) and the locally recommended interventions but data lacking on the Country's use of BBE for Tungiasis Control and elimination. There is a need to develop a training manual, IEC Materials, and Community/Civil Societies Organizations Materials for sensitizations to support those affected and the need for integrated coordinated community disease surveillance mechanisms with a comprehensive approach. Vector-Borne and Neglected Tropical Disease control division will be critical in providing solutions to this problem.

6. Recommendations

It is therefore suggested that countrywide studies are required to establish the exact prevalence and magnitude of Tungiasis infections in Uganda, assessing the epidemiological, socio-cultural context, behavioral and ecological risk factors. There is a need to assess the impact on school-age children (SAC) attendance 5–14 years and the disability-adjusted life years associated with the infections.

Acknowledgements

The authors would like to thank in particular the research assistants who were involved in the data collection. We are also grateful for the contribution of District NTD focal Persons for their efforts in mobilizing the communities for the study. Approval for the surveys was gratefully received from the Ethics committee of the Virtual University of Uganda (VUU-PGDPH-2016-037) and Vector Control Division Research Ethics (VCDREC/090) and Uganda National Council of Science & Technology (UNCST). Individuals who participated in the study provided written consent and assent before the study took place.

Authors contributions

Conceptualization, Data curation, Formal analysis, Funding acquisition, Methodology, Project administration, Visualization, Writing – original draft, Writing – review & editing all by the author.

Funding

This study was a student lead study supported by primary healthcare funds from the Ministry of Health, Republic of Uganda.

Conflict of interest

The authors declare no conflict of interest.

Author details

Moses Adriko[1,2,3,4]

1 Vector Control Division, Ministry of Health, Kampala, Uganda

2 Uganda Institute of Allied Health and Management Science (UIAHMS), School of Medical Entomology and Parasitology, Kampala, Uganda

3 Ministry of Health, Kampala, Uganda

4 The Virtual University, Uganda, Kampala, Uganda

*Address all correspondence to: adrikomoses@gmail.com

References

[1] Eisele M, Heukelbach J, Van Marck E, Mehlhorn H, Meckes O, Franck S, et al. Investigations on the biology, epidemiology, pathology and control of Tunga penetrans in Brazil: I. Natural history of tungiasis in man. Parasitology Research. 2003;**90**(2):87-99

[2] Veraldi S, Valsecchi M. Imported tungiasis: A report of 19 cases and review of the literature. International Journal of Dermatology. 2007;**46**(10):1061-1066

[3] Vaira F, Nazzaro G, Veraldi S. Tungiasis: "the greatest curse that has ever afflicted Africa". JAMA Dermatology. 2014;**150**(7):708

[4] Ade-Serrano M, Ejezie GC. Prevalence of tungiasis in Oto-Ijanikin village, Badagry, Lagos State, Nigeria. Annals of Tropical Medicine and Parasitology. 1981;**75**(4):471-472

[5] Nte A, Eke F. Jigger infestation in children in a rural area of Rivers State of Nigeria. West African Journal of Medicine. 1995;**14**(1):56-58

[6] Carvalho RWd, Almeida ABd, Barbosa-Silva SC, Amorim M, Ribeiro PC, Serra-Freire NM. The patterns of tungiasis in Araruama township, state of Rio de Janeiro, Brazil. Memórias do Instituto Oswaldo Cruz. 2003;**98**(1):31-36

[7] Heukelbach J, Franck S, Feldmeier H. Therapy of tungiasis: A double-blinded randomized controlled trial with oral ivermectin. Memórias do Instituto Oswaldo Cruz. 2004;**99**(8):873-876

[8] Ugbomoiko US, Ofoezie IE, Heukelbach J. Tungiasis: High prevalence, parasite load, and morbidity in a rural community in Lagos State, Nigeria. International Journal of Dermatology. 2007;**46**(5):475-481

[9] Heukelbach J, Jackson A, Ariza L, Calheiros C, Soares V, Feldmeier H. Epidemiology and clinical aspects of tungiasis (sand flea infestation) in Alagoas State, Brazil. Journal of Infection in Developing Countries. 2007;**1**:202-209

[10] Sachse MM, Guldbakke KK, Khachemoune A. Tunga penetrans: A stowaway from around the world. Journal of the European Academy of Dermatology and Venereology. 2007;**21**(1):11-16

[11] Thielecke M, Feldmeier H. The fate of the embedded virgin sand flea Tunga penetrans: Hypothesis, self-experimentation and photographic sequence. Travel Medicine and Infectious Disease. 2013;**11**(6):440-443

[12] Ugbomoiko US, Ariza L, Heukelbach J. Pigs are the most important animal reservoir for Tunga penetrans (jigger flea) in rural Nigeria. Tropical Doctor. 2008;**38**(4):226-227

[13] Kehr JD, Heukelbach J, Mehlhorn H, Feldmeier H. Morbidity assessment in sand flea disease (tungiasis). Parasitology Research. 2007;**100**(2):413-421

[14] Sentongo E, Wabinga H. Tungiasis presenting as a soft tissue oral lesion. BMC Oral Health. 2014;**14**:112

[15] Jawoko K. Jiggers outbreak in Uganda. CMAJ. 2011;**183**(1):E33-E34

[16] Hotez PJ, Bottazzi ME, Franco-Paredes C, Ault SK, Periago MR. The neglected tropical diseases of Latin America and the Caribbean: A review of disease burden and distribution and a roadmap for control and elimination.

PLoS Neglected Tropical Diseases. 2008;**2**(9):e300

[17] Feldmeier H, Eisele M, Van Marck E, Mehlhorn H, Ribeiro R, Heukelbach J. Investigations on the biology, epidemiology, pathology and control of Tunga penetrans in Brazil: IV. Clinical and histopathology. Parasitol Res. 2004;**94**(4):275-282

[18] Pilger D, Schwalfenberg S, Heukelbach J, Witt L, Mehlhorn H, Mencke N, et al. Investigations on the biology, epidemiology, pathology, and control of Tunga penetrans in Brazil: VII. The importance of animal reservoirs for human infestation. Parasitology Research. 2008;**102**(5):875-880

[19] Pampiglione S, Trentini M, Fioravanti ML, Onore G, Rivasi F. On a new species of sand flea from Ecuador and tungiasis, a problem of Public Health in many developing countries. Annali di Igiene. 2003;**15**(5):747-752

[20] Clyti E, Couppie P, Deligny C, Jouary T, Sainte-Marie D, Pradinaud R. Effectiveness of 20% salicylated vaseline in the treatment of profuse tungiasis. Report of 8 cases in French Guiana. Bulletin de la Societe de pathologie exotique. 2003;**96**(5):412-414

[21] Mutebi F, Krucken J, Mencke N, Feldmeier H, von Samson-Himmelstjerna G, Waiswa C. Two severe cases of Tungiasis in Goat Kids in Uganda. Journal of Insect Science. 2016;**16**

[22] Mutebi F, Krucken J, Feldmeier H, Waiswa C, Mencke N, von Samson-Himmelstjerna G. Tungiasis-associated morbidity in pigs and dogs in endemic villages of Uganda. Parasites & Vectors. 2016;**9**:44

[23] MOH. Uganda Master Plan for National Neglected Tropical Diseases Programmes: 2017-2022. 2017

[24] Mutebi F, Krucken J, Feldmeier H, Waiswa C, Mencke N, Sentongo E, et al. Animal reservoirs of zoonotic Tungiasis in Endemic Rural Villages of Uganda. PLoS Neglected Tropical Diseases. 2015;**9**(10):e0004126

[25] Mutebi F, Krucken J, von Samson-Himmelstjerna G, Waiswa C, Mencke N, Eneku W, et al. Animal and human tungiasis-related knowledge and treatment practices among animal keeping households in Bugiri District, South-Eastern Uganda. Acta Tropica. 2018;**177**:81-88

[26] Muehlen M, Heukelbach J, Wilcke T, Winter B, Mehlhorn H, Feldmeier H. Investigations on the biology, epidemiology, pathology and control of Tunga penetrans in Brazil. II. Prevalence, parasite load and topographic distribution of lesions in the population of a traditional fishing village. Parasitology Research. 2003;**90**(6):449-455

[27] Wafula ST, Ssemugabo C, Namuhani N, Musoke D, Ssempebwa J, Halage AA. Prevalence and risk factors associated with tungiasis in Mayuge district, Eastern Uganda. The Pan African Medical Journal. 2016;**24**:77

[28] Mutebi F, von Samson-Himmelstjerna G, Feldmeier H, Waiswa C, Bukeka Muhindo J, Krucken J. Successful treatment of severe tungiasis in pigs using a topical aerosol containing chlorfenvinphos, dichlorphos and gentian violet. PLoS Neglected Tropical Diseases. 2016;**10**(10):e0005056

[29] Mutebi F, Krucken J, Feldmeier H, Waiswa C, Mencke N, Eneku W, et al. High intensity of Tunga penetrans infection causing severe disease among pigs in Busoga, South Eastern Uganda. BMC Veterinary Research. 2017;**13**(1):206

[30] Ugbomoiko US, Ariza L, Ofoezie IE, Heukelbach J. Risk factors for tungiasis in Nigeria: Identification of targets for effective intervention. PLoS Neglected Tropical Diseases. 2007;**1**(3):e87

[31] Muehlen M, Feldmeier H, Wilcke T, Winter B, Heukelbach J. Identifying risk factors for tungiasis and heavy infestation in a resource-poor community in northeast Brazil. Transactions of the Royal Society of Tropical Medicine and Hygiene. 2006;**100**(4):371-380

[32] Ugbomoiko US, Ariza L, Babamale AO, Heukelbach J. Prevalence and clinical aspects of tungiasis in south-west Nigerian schoolchildren. Tropical Doctor. 2017;**47**(1):34-38

[33] Klimpel S, Mehlhorn H, Heukelbach J, Feldmeier H, Mencke N. Field trial of the efficacy of a combination of imidacloprid and permethrin against Tunga penetrans (sand flea, jigger flea) in dogs in Brazil. Parasitology Research. 2005;**97** (Suppl. 1):S113-S1S9

[34] Heukelbach J, Costa AM, Wilcke T, Mencke N, Feldmeier H. The animal reservoir of Tunga penetrans in severely affected communities of north-east Brazil. Medical and Veterinary Entomology. 2004;**18**(4):329-335

[35] Wiese S, Elson L, Reichert F, Mambo B, Feldmeier H. Prevalence, intensity and risk factors of tungiasis in Kilifi County, Kenya: I. Results from a community-based study. PLoS Neglected Tropical Diseases. 2017;**11**(10):e0005925

[36] Nyangacha RM, Odongo D, Oyieke F, Ochwoto M, Korir R, Ngetich RK, et al. Secondary bacterial infections and antibiotic resistance among tungiasis patients in Western, Kenya. PLoS Neglected Tropical Diseases. 2017;**11**(9):e0005901

Chapter 7

Exosomes Therapy in Zoonoses

Fernando Ojeda, Gabriela Barreto and Sinforiano J. Posadas

Abstract

Exosomes are smaller extracellular vesicles (EVs) involved in complex intercellular communication, which were first discovered in sheep reticulocytes. Exosomes include two subpopulations, large (Exo-L, 90–120 nm) and small (Exo-S, 60–80 nm) exosome vesicles. Recently studies of RNA viruses including SARS-CoV-2 have demonstrated that exosomes release regulatory factors from infected cells and deliver other functional host genetic elements to neighbouring cells, and these functions are involved in the infection process and modulate the cellular responses. This review provides an overview of the biogenesis, composition, and some of the most striking functions of exosome secretion in zoonoses and identifies physiological/pathological areas in need of further research as well as potential therapeutic agents in zoonotic disease.

Keywords: RNA virus, exosome, infection, miRNA, active proteins, lipids, and nucleic acids

1. Introduction

Zoonotic diseases are estimated to cause 60% of infections in humans. Treatments are mainly based on the use of antibiotics and antimicrobials; this creates resistant strains, searching for new therapeutic approaches of paramount importance [1]. Cell-based therapy, and especially stem cell therapy, has become a promising therapeutic field in which many see opportunities to treat incurable diseases. Among the various cell types, MSCs have attracted attention due to the source of origin, a high proliferation rate, low-invasive and ethically unproblematic procurement procedure [2].

The therapeutic effect of MSCs seems to rely on the modifications they exert on their microenvironment through paracrine interactions, secretion of soluble factors, cytokines, and trophic factors. It is possible to simplify treatment by using only the components secreted by MSCs, constituting the so-called secretome, which includes immunoregulatory factors (e.g., IL-6 and IL-10), prostaglandin E2, hepatocyte growth factor, indolamine 2,3-dioxygenase, nitric oxide, TGF-ß, and human leukocyte antigen, as well as extracellular vesicles. In fact, these cells can be considered potent pharmacotherapeutics that release biologically active substances [3].

Once released, EVs and soluble proteins interact with target cells (by ligand-receptor interaction or by internalisation) and modulate cellular responses. The secretome can activate endogenous stem cells and progenitor cells, suppress apoptosis, regulate the inflammatory response, stimulate extracellular matrix remodelling and angiogenesis, reduce fibrosis and mediate chemoattraction [4].

Exosomes are nanoscale extracellular vesicles with a lipid bilayer of endocytic origin and are secreted by almost all cell types and physiological states [5]. They are small with a diameter of 40–100 nm [6] and can be permeable to biological barriers.

Exosome formation takes place by internal plasma membrane budding to form multivesicular bodies (MVB) [7], which can also originate from the trans-Golgi network [8]. Within the MVB, exosomes are formed by further internal budding and then released by fusion of the MVB membrane with the plasma membrane [9].

Exosomes contain a large number of parental cell proteins, and their membrane is abundant with proteins of the tetraspanin family (CD9, CD63, CD81, and CD82), which are widely used as exosome markers. They also have adhesion surface proteins to facilitate their internalisation by other cells [10].

They have a defined composition, depending on cell type, pathology, and activation state, thus exerting their role on specific target cells to release their protein content, mRNA, and, importantly, specific microRNA molecules [11].

Exosomes are considered safe because they lack the potential for endogenous tumor formation as they cannot self-replicate, have low immunogenicity and, when injected intravenously, lead to low embolism formation [12]. The application of exosomes in therapy also has technological advantages: they can be managed and stored easily, and they are a suitable product for use in emergency interventions [13].

Exosomes can be isolated from cell culture supernatant by different methods (each with different limitations). Current techniques are based on exosome size (30–100 nm), density (1.13–1.21 g/ml), and exosome-specific markers (such as CD63). The general method is based on ultracentrifugation of the cell culture supernatant. However, this method often entrains impurities from microvesicles or other cellular detritus. In addition, the high centrifugal force and duration of centrifugation can cause damage to the exosomes [14].

Summarising, with a conglomerate of cytokines, growth factors, mRNAs, and microRNAs having anti-inflammatory, immunomodulatory and regenerative functions; exosomes play a role as paracrine and endocrine mediators; a fact that, together with their safety profile, stability, and scalability, make them a valuable treatment option for zoonotic diseases either as vehicles or as vaccines themselves (see **Table 1**) [15].

In view of the above, the objectives of this chapter are as follows:

1. To review zoonotic diseases of public health importance, as well as their current treatments.

2. To evaluate the therapeutic capacity of exosomes in infections of zoonotic origin.

    a. Possibility of altering target cells by acting as molecules in intercellular communication.

    b. Potential to act as a vehicle for the delivery of desired therapeutical targets.

2. Methodology

The study presented here follows a qualitative methodology, as it pursues the description and interpretative understanding of exosome therapy for diseases of zoonotic origin. Specifically, we will stick to documentary research to approach the aforementioned object of study. Thus, both review and research articles, as

Pathogen type	Pathogen	Role of exosome	What causes	Reference
Virus	Rabie	Intercellular communication	Viral infection process	[16]
		Vehicle	Bind acetylcholine receptor	[17–19]
		Intercellular communication	Inhibit replication and actívate immune system	[20]
	Ebola	Intercellular communication	Cell death and apoptosis	[21, 22]
		Vehicle	Increase in the levels of cytotoxic T-lymphocyte response	[23]
	HIV	Vehicle	Viral suppression	[24]
		Vehicle	Reactivation of HIV-infected CD4 T cells	[25]
	SARS-CoV-2	Intercellular communication	General improvement of the body	[26–28]
		Vehicle	General improvement of the body	[29]
		Intercellular communication	Nervous system recovery	[30–32]
	Influenza	Vehicle	That virus replication inhibited	[33]
		Intercellular communication	Release of pro-inflammatory cytokines and the overexpression of type I interferon	[34]
		Intercellular communication	Restore the permeability lung epithelial	[35]
Bacteria	Brucella	Vehicle	Immune response	[36, 37]
		Intercellular communication	Enhance immune system response	[38]
	Salmonella	Intercellular communication	Inflammatory reaction	[39]
		Intercellular communication	Innate and adaptive response	[40]
	M. tuberculosis	vehicle and adjuvant	Intensify the immune response	[41, 42]
		Intercellular communication	Exert an immune response via Th1 and Th2	[43]
Parasite	*T. gondii*	Intercellular communication	Response Th1 secrete IL-2 and IFN-gamma, activate macrophages and NK cells	[44]
		Intercellular communication	It increases fertility and this is because the immune response is type 2	[45]

Fungi	*C. neoformans*	Intercellular communication	Complement system is activated, leading to inflammation, phagocytosis and cell lysis	[46]
		Intercellular communication	Immune response	[47]

This table describes the pathogens and their origin, as well as the function of exosomes in the organism. Source: Compilation based.

Table 1.
Overview of the different pathogens and how exosomes work as therapy.

well as governmental websites will be used. In all cases, the types of documents are electronic. As this is documentary research of an exploratory nature, the aim of this exploratory documentary research is fitting the above-mentioned objectives.

The studies have been reviewed in different databases:

- Google Scholar: Google's tool for finding books and journals, bibliographic references with abstracts, full texts, or personal and institutional websites.
- PubMed: digital storage system that integrates biomedical scientific journals, with access to abstracts, bibliographic references, tables and figures or complete articles.
- medRxiv/bioRxiv: search engines that allow for the consultation of unpublished scientific articles in the health field that are not peer-reviewed.
- WHO website: because it is the specialised body in charge of management, prevention, and decision-making in the field of global health issues.
- Website of the Spanish government: for consultation of updated COVID-19 data to updated COVID-19 data at the global level.

The search for documents was carried out based on keywords such as zoonosis, exosome, vaccine, infection, intercellular communication, rabies, Ebola, HIV, SARS-CoV-2, influenza, brucella, salmonella, mycobacterium tuberculosis, toxoplasma gondii, and cryptococcus neoformans.

For the development of the documentary work, a total of 108 bibliographic sources were found, based on: (1) year of publication, except for the study by Pan BT (1985), and (2) relevance of the study associated with our objectives, as some of them, despite addressing the subject, did so from a more general perspective.

For all these reasons, the sample includes information of both a qualitative and quantitative nature, which allows us to have a bigger knowledge range to argue properly our work.

3. Exosome-based therapy for zoonotic diseases

3.1 Rabies

Rabies virus is a single-stranded RNA belonging to the Rhabdovirus family. They are bullet-shaped, with a flat and a rounded end, an envelope with spicules surrounding the genome, and a helical capsid. The Rhabdovirus family includes the genus Vesiculovirus, which causes vesicular stomatitis virus, and the genus Lyssavirus, which causes rabies [48].

The receptor of the rabies virus is the nicotinic acetylcholine receptor. It enters the cell by endocytosis and replication takes place in the cytoplasm. It has RNA-dependent RNA polymerase. Transcription of the viral RNA produces five individual mRNAs that will give rise to five proteins, a process that takes place in the Negri corpuscles. Negri bodies are cytoplasmic inclusion bodies that correspond to aggregates of viral nucleocapsids and are formed as a result of the replication process (diagnostically useful) [49, 50].

Rabies is a zoonosis whose reservoir is wild animals, mainly bats, and dogs (in 99% of cases) [48]. The virus is excreted in the saliva of an infected animal and enters other animals through bite wounds or scratches. The virus is very labile, so transmission through contaminated objects is rare. Human-to-human transmission is not confirmed [51].

Pre-exposure prophylaxis is based on an inactivated vaccine in at-risk personnel. As the incubation period is long, post-exposure vaccination is feasible. The original vaccine designed by Pasteur was an attenuated virus vaccine (obtained from neural tissue of infected animals) and had the disadvantage of producing adverse reactions with allergic encephalomyelitis. Post-exposure prophylaxis is based on wound lavage, passive immunisation with human rabies immune globulin and active immunisation with inactivated vaccine (five intramuscular doses) [52].

It is known that infected cells release exosomes into the environment [53, 54]; however, the role of exosomes in infections is not entirely clear. Therefore, Wang et al. evaluated the role of exosomes in rabies virus infection. After isolation of exosomes by density gradient, they characterised them by transmission electron microscopy and western blotting. The results were that, after infection, the release of exosomes increased. They also used treatment with two inhibitors of exosome secretion, GW4869, and si-Rab27a, and found not only that exosome secretion decreased, but also that the presence of intra- and extracellular viral RNA was reduced. This finding provides a better understanding of the role of exosomes in rabies virus infection and proposes it as a new research target for the development of therapeutic strategies [16].

Research groups such as Yang et al., Alvarez-Erviti et al. and Kumar et al. highlight the role of rabies virus glycoprotein-modified exosomes (RVG-modified exosomes) for, in addition to being loaded with the desired content to tackle the condition, the ability to cross the blood-brain barrier and bind specifically to the acetylcholine receptor of neurons [17–19].

Yang et al. conducted a study with the human diploid cell line Medical Research Council-5 (MRC-5), which is used to develop vaccines. In the case of rabies, a vaccine based on this cell line exists, but with low efficacy due to the limitation of infection on the cells. These researchers demonstrated that, following rabies virus infection in the MRC-5 cell line, exosomes have a dual function: (I) to interfere with the type I interferon signalling pathway to increase its production and (II) through this regulation, to inhibit rabies virus replication [20].

3.2 Ebola

Ebola virus is a filamentous, enveloped, helical nucleocapsid, single-stranded negative RNA genome. It belongs to the Filovirus family where the Marburg virus is also found. The genome has the information to encode seven structural proteins that form the virion. It replicates in the cytoplasm similar to Rhabdoviruses [55].

The Ebola disease outbreak in West Africa, which began in March 2014, was the largest viral haemorrhagic epidemic in history. Nearly 40% of people who contracted Ebola during this outbreak died. The natural reservoir is unknown. Transmission is by direct contact with infected blood and secretions; there is no airborne transmission. There is no vaccine or specific treatment. Favipiravir, an antiviral against RNA viruses, has been used; in addition, passive immunisation is carried out by the administration of sera [56].

Exosomes released by the Ebola virus, called VP40+, cause cell death and apoptosis, eventually destroying immune cells [21]. Because exosomes play a role in intercellular communication and influence cellular responses, they may be targeted for therapy development, specifically for vaccine production [22].

CD8 T cells play a central role in antiviral immunity and are also involved in the immune response generated against other intracellular pathogens, such as intracellular bacteria. Destruction of virus-infected cells requires the T-lymphocyte receptor to recognise peptides associated with MHC class I molecules. This triggers the activation of lymphocytes to (I) destroy infected cells and (II) produce inflammatory cytokines [57]. This immune response has been seen in Ebola survivors [58] and in non-human primates [59].

Exosomes are vesicles released by all cell types of the organism [60, 61]. By developing intramuscular DNA vector vaccines, namely NEFmut, scientists Anticoli S. *et al*. incorporated exosomes to study the immune response against Ebola virus (based on those discussed above). They were able to see an increase in the levels of cytotoxic T-lymphocyte response and cope with the disease [23].

3.3 HIV

Human Immunodeficiency Virus (HIV) belongs to the retrovirus family. It is a virus with two identical single-stranded RNA molecules enveloped. They are called *Retroviridae* because they possess an enzyme with reverse transcriptase activity (retrotranscriptase) that allows RNA to be transcribed into DNA, making it an RNA-dependent DNA polymerase. There are four families of retroviruses: oncornavirus (human T-lymphotropic virus), spumavirus (only in animals), alpharetrovirus (Rous sarcoma virus), and lentivirus (HIV) [62].

Replication begins with the binding of viral glycoproteins to the primary receptor, the CD4 molecule, and to the co-receptors CCR5 or CXCR4. They infect CD4 T cells and other cells that express the CD4 molecule on their surface, such as monocytes, macrophages, or dendritic cells. They penetrate the host cell by fusion of the envelope with the cell membrane. Binding to the co-receptor brings the envelope into contact with the plasma membrane and the glycoprotein gp41 promotes membrane fusion. The genome is released into the cytoplasm and undergoes a reverse transcription process, which uses the transfer RNA as a primer [63].

To avoid the development of HIV resistance, a combination of three drugs from two different classes is recommended. The recommended antiretroviral treatment in naïve patients (those who have not had previous antiretroviral treatment) is outlined below [64, 65]:

- 2 NRTIs (nucleoside reverse transcriptase inhibitors) + 1 NNRTI (non-nucleoside reverse transcriptase inhibitor).
- 2 NRTIs (nucleoside reverse transcriptase inhibitors) + 1 PI (protease inhibitor).

- 2 NRTIs (nucleoside reverse transcriptase inhibitors) + 1 INI (integrase inhibitor).

The above-mentioned therapy has side effects such as decreased life expectancy and the virus may develop resistance. Shrivastava et al. developed an HIV promoter targeting the ZPZ-362 protein that fuses with DNA methyltransferase domains capable of long-term HIV suppression. This promoter is introduced into exosomes acting as a transport medium and allowing delivery to act in epigenetic regulation. Analysing the results, they found that this transport medium performed its function perfectly, as once inside, the methylation machinery acted, leading to viral suppression [24].

More than half of HIV-infected people suffer from cognitive problems due to prolonged inflammation and disruption of the blood-brain barrier (BBB). The problem is that not all treatments are able to cross the BBB. Therefore, exosomes have been proposed as drug delivery vehicles since, among their many characteristics, is the ability to cross the BBB [66].

Among the essential genes for viral replication that form a regulatory protein is Tat (Trans-Activator of Transcription). It increases the level of HIV double-stranded RNA transcription; in its absence, there is little RNA transcription. On this premise, Tang et al. introduced the Tat protein into exosomes, enabling the reactivation of HIV-infected CD4 T cells. This makes it possible to deal with latently infected cells [25].

3.4 SARS-CoV-2

SARS-CoV-2 belongs to the coronavirus (CoV) family, named after its characteristic morphology, which resembles a solar corona when viewed under the electron microscope. CoVs are classified into four different genera according to their phylogeny and genomic structure: alpha, beta, gamma, and delta [67]. They are a family of viruses that can cause multiple systemic infections or damage in various animal species [68]. Genomic analyses show that SARS-CoV-2 is from the same beta coronavirus (βCoV) family as SARS-CoV-1 and Middle East respiratory syndrome coronavirus (MERS-CoV), and they have high sequence homology [69]. In 2003 SARS-CoV-1 caused an epidemic with 8273 cases and 775 deaths [70]. The MERS-CoV epidemic, however, caused 1139 cases and 431 deaths in 2013 [71].

Coronaviruses are composed of a single-stranded positive-sense RNA, with a genome ranging from 26.2 to 31.7 kb [67]. It has mainly three viral proteins in the virion envelope: spike protein (S), membrane protein (M), and envelope protein (E). The spike protein mediates virus entry and determines the range of potential hosts, cell tropism, and pathogenic disease [72].

SARS-CoV-2 uses angiotensin-converting enzyme 2 (ACE2) as a receptor to infect bronchial epithelial ciliated cells and type II pneumocytes [73], which explains the severity of lung involvement. In addition to the lungs, the receptor is widely distributed in the gastrointestinal, hepatic, renal, nervous, cardiovascular, and other systems. This can lead to pathologies beyond the respiratory system [74]. After binding to the receptor, the viruses fuse their envelope with the host cell membrane and the nucleocapsids reach the target cell [75].

At the end of 2019, several cases of acute respiratory infection were discovered in the Chinese province of Wuhan. Those affected had in common pneumonia of unknown aetiology and exposure to the Wuhan market [76]. Due to its virological similarity and clinical picture with Severe Acute Respiratory Syndrome (SARS) caused by the SARS-CoV-1 coronavirus, the World Health Organisation (WHO) named the coronavirus SARS-CoV-2 and the disease it causes COVID-19 [77].

On 11 March 2020, the WHO declared the disease a pandemic because of the increase in the number of people affected since the discovery of the virus [78]. At the time of writing (25 March 2022) and according to the Ministry of Health, the total number of COVID-19 cases worldwide is 47,465,969,674 [79], affecting more than 200 countries. It has therefore become a global health problem and many researchers are currently seeking to eradicate it.

Fortunately, scientists have succeeded in developing vaccines to tackle COVID-19. These are composed of mRNA or adenoviral vectors that encode the virus and are enveloped by lipids [80]. Millions of lives have been saved thanks to these vaccines, but issues such as the use of booster doses, the origin of SARS-CoV-2 variants, and whether the vaccines can cope with the side effects of the disease remain unresolved.

Multiple preclinical studies have demonstrated favourable therapeutic effects of intravenously administered MSC-derived exosomes in animal models of acute lung injury [26], acute respiratory distress syndrome (ARDS) [27], asthma, and other inflammatory diseases, with analyses revealing reduced alveolar inflammation, enhanced oedema clearance, restoration of permeable epithelium, membranes and other sequelae of cytokine storm (**Figure 1**) [28].

Taking advantage of the benefits provided by exosomes, scientists Jiang et al. studied the feasibility of an exosome-based vaccine. They introduced the spike protein-binding domain into *Salmonella typhimurium* exosomes. Once the animals

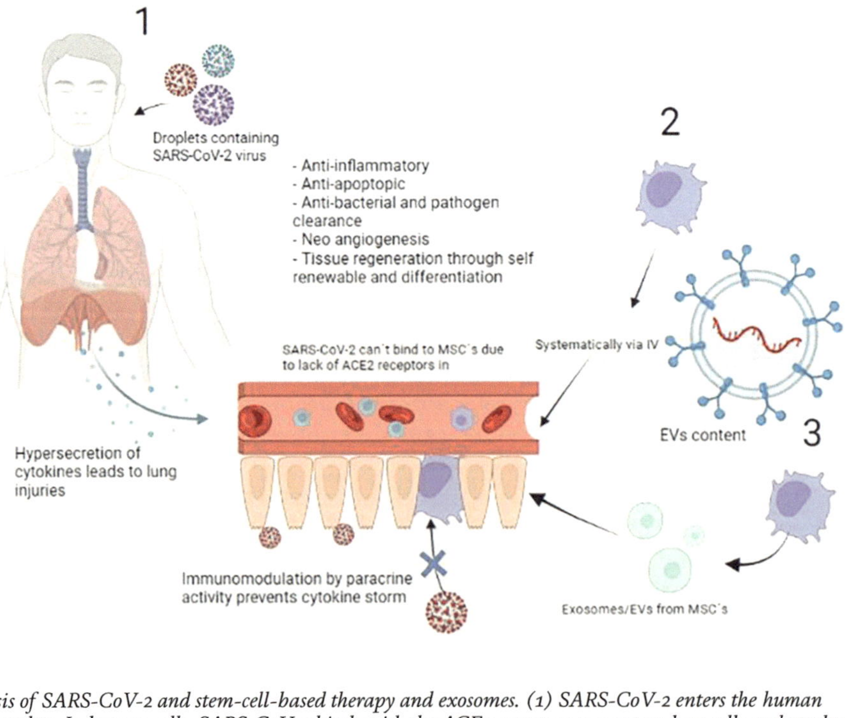

Figure 1.
Pathogenesis of SARS-CoV-2 and stem-cell-based therapy and exosomes. (1) SARS-CoV-2 enters the human body via droplets. In human cells, SARS-CoV-2 binds with the ACE2 receptors present on host cells and produces a cytokine storm. This storm results in a severe lung injury. (2) MSCs. (3) MSCs-Exo or EVs are considered a possible future treatment due to many of their properties, such as ACE2—(lack of ACE2 receptors) which prevents a cytokine storm and immune modulation and restoration of damaged cells due to their essential growth factors and metabolites. Source: Compilation based.

were vaccinated (first group), they tested the control group (unvaccinated animals infected with the Delta variant). The first group had less virus replication, less alveolar damage, a slight or no decrease in body mass, and a high titre of IgG antibodies measured in serum and bronchoalveolar lavage compared to the control. This demonstrates the feasibility of an exosome-based vaccine against COVID-19 [29].

One of the side effects of COVID-19 is how it can affect the nervous system. There are several reasons for this. First, because of the cytokine storm producing neuroinflammation which is the basis of numerous neurological diseases such as Alzheimer's, Parkinson's, multiple sclerosis [30], or even psychiatric conditions [31]. Secondly, the direct neuroinvasive capacity of ACE2 receptors, which are also found in the nervous system and are considered potential targets [32]. The third is the indirect action on the nervous system due to the already demonstrated relationship between the intestinal microbiota and the nervous system, as the virus invades the intestinal mucosa and causes inflammatory processes that can lead to neurological damage [31]. Therefore, exosomes could be used as a therapy for this side effect, as intranasal administration not only offers the benefits mentioned above but is also a direct route of entry into the nervous system and also has the ability to cross the blood-brain barrier [29].

3.5 Influenza

The Orthomyxovirus family has a helical capsid, is enveloped and the negative single-stranded RNA is segmented into eight fragments. Influenza viruses or influenza viruses stand out. There are three types: A, the most important; B, the endemic type; C, very rare [81].

The influenza virus transcribes and replicates its genome in the nucleus of the target cell. Replication begins with the binding of haemagglutinin to the sialic acid of cell surface glycoproteins. They replicate in the nucleus because they cannot synthesise their own mRNA. Transcriptase uses cellular RNA as a primer to initiate viral mRNA synthesis (cap-snatching) [82]. The mRNA is synthesised using 5′-CAP ends of heterologous nuclear RNA as a primer (mRNA cap-stealing). It is assembled in the cytoplasm and exits by budding through the plasma membrane [83].

Virus transmission is airborne via respiratory secretions. Its genetic diversity is based on its segmented genome structure and its ability to infect and replicate in humans and many animal species, such as birds and pigs. Influenza virus type A is characterised by high antigenic variability, much higher than in type B and C [84].

Antigenic variations can be of two types:

- Most commonly, minor changes (antigenic drifts, antigenic drift, or antigenic slippage), involve a change in the surrounding strain within the same virus type. They are due to point mutations in haemagglutinin and neuraminidase. They are responsible for epidemics [85].

- Major changes (antigenic shifts, antigenic jumping, or antigenic conversion) show a change in the surrounding virus subtype and are responsible for periodic influenza A virus pandemics. This antigenic shift occurs due to the exchange between the gene segments of different influenza virus strains (both human and animal) when the two strains infect the same cell. Such recombination only occurs in the pig and occurs between human and avian viruses. It should be noted that this process only occurs in influenza A virus [85].

For at-risk personnel, possible immunoprophylaxis is a vaccination with inactivated viruses. Other therapeutic options include amantadine, oseltamivir, and zanamivir, which should be administered early within 48 h of symptom onset [81].

miRNAs are single-stranded RNAs that are approximately 22 nucleotides in length and have the ability to regulate the expression of various genes that play a role in development, cancer, defence against organisms, immunity, homeostasis, etc. Scientists Liu et al. studied the role of miRNAs in influenza virus, focusing their research on the functional role of hsa-miR-1975 in the defence of the infected organism. The methodology was based on assessing the antiviral effects of this miRNA by RT-PCR, Western Blot, and plaque assays. The results obtained were not only that virus replication is inhibited, but also that the release of hsa-miR-1975 occurs via exosomes [33]. This indicates evidence of the importance of investigating the therapeutic possibilities of exosomes due to their ability to harbour content that modifies cellular communication [10].

One notable function of exosomes is in cell-cell communication in the immune system, aiding the body's defence against pathogens. Exosomes carry proteins, and mRNA and, as mentioned above, can carry miRNA. An investigation was carried out to look at the performance of exosomes against influenza virus infection. Among the miRNAs studied, miR-483-3p emphasised its role in defense. The researchers were able to demonstrate its capabilities in the release of pro-inflammatory cytokines and the overexpression of type I interferon. They were able to demonstrate the role of exosomes in the inflammatory reaction when a microorganism is present in the body [34].

Influenza virus is acquired via the respiratory tract through inhalation of aerosolized viral particles. Initially, local infection of the upper respiratory tract is established and can lead to acute lung injury. MSCs, specifically umbilical cord-derived MSCs (UC-MSCs) and their derived exosomes, which mediate paracrine transport, have the ability to restore the lung microenvironment. They restore the permeability that characterises lung epithelial cells and removes alveolar fluid from impaired cells [35].

3.6 Brucella

The most clinically relevant species are *Brucella abortus*, *Brucella melitensis*, and *Brucella suis*. They are responsible for classical zoonoses and the most prominent reservoirs are cattle and wild animals; cows (*B. abortus*), goats (*B. melitensis*), and pigs (*B. suis*) [86]. The zoonosis in humans is known as brucellosis, Bang's disease, Malta fever, or undulant fever [87].

They are Gram- coccobacilli, non-flagellating (hence not motile). They grow only under aerobic conditions, and are non-fermenting and slow-growing. They are facultative intracellular pathogens [88].

Brucellosis is a globally distributed zoonosis, is an occupational disease, and is a reportable disease in most countries of the world. *B. melitensis* infections are more frequent in Mediterranean countries, Latin America and Asia. The main prophylactic measure is to avoid exposure and prevent consumption of unpasteurised dairy products. Isolation of infected persons is not necessary, as the infection is not transmitted from person to person [87].

Attenuated *B. abortus* and melitensis vaccines have been successful in preventing infection in cattle [88]. The absence of an effective human vaccine is a cause for concern, because Brucella could be used as an agent of biological terrorism. Current treatment in humans is based on doxycycline with streptomycin or gentamicin; the alternative is co-trimoxazole. Antibiotic therapy should be prolonged for 3–4 weeks. For children and pregnant women, co-trimoxazole and rifampicin are used [87].

As mentioned above, exosomes can function as vehicles and deliver various molecules. This ability is exploited by macrophages to transport interferon-induced transmembrane protein 3 (IFITM3) from uninfected to infected macrophages once the organism is exposed to the Brucella pathogen [36]. IFITM3 is a critical protein for the immune system as it prevents the replication of foreign agents when they enter the body [37]. In this study by Yi et al., they found, in addition to the transmembrane protein mentioned above, that exosomes transport multiple proteins after infection including those involved in the immune response. This ability of exosomes represents a breakthrough in the development of a vaccine to tackle brucellosis [36].

In the research and development of an effective vaccine for Malta fever, a group of scientists led by Solanki KS treated mice inoculated with a virulent strain of *B. abortus* S544 with exosomes. The exosomes were outer membrane vesicles extracted from *B. abortus* S19Δper an attenuated strain, OMVs S19 Δper. After analysis of the results and comparison between the control group (inoculated with the strain, but not treated) and the vaccinated group (inoculated with the strain and vaccinated with OMVs S19) they were able to conclude that there was an increase in the Th1 and Th2 immune system response, with an increase in IgG antibody titres, and cytokines such as IL-2, IL-4, TNF, among others [38].

3.7 Salmonella

Typhoid salmonellosis is caused by *Salmonella typhi* and *Salmonella paratyphi* serotypes A, B, and C. S. typhi has a capsular antigen that does not form a true capsule because it does not completely cover the cell wall. Adherence of the bacteria to jejunal cells (M cells) facilitates invasion by endocytosis-transfer-exocytosis. Dissemination via blood and lymph from the intestinal tract occurs. Cases of typhoid salmonellosis in Europe are imported by travellers and occur as a circumstantial epidemic. Humans are the only reservoir; they can survive in the gallbladder, generating asymptomatic carriers [89, 90].

Enteric salmonellosis is caused by *Salmonella enteritidis* and *Salmonella typhimurium*. The bacteria gain access to the gastrointestinal tract through food (animal reservoir). Adhesion to enterocytes of the ileum and colon facilitates mucosal invasion mediated by bacterial surface invasions. Endotoxin production is the main cause of food-borne toxic-infection. Enteric salmonellosis occurs both endemically and epidemically. The main focus of infection is livestock; it is a zoonosis [91, 92].

Typhoidal salmonellosis should be treated with antibiotics. Third-generation cephalosporins are recommended. Other antibiotics such as ciprofloxacin or co-trimoxazole may be treatment alternatives. In typhoid salmonellosis, elimination of chronic carriers presents a problem but can be achieved with high doses of antibiotics (4-quinolones or ampicillin) [89, 93].

In enteric salmonellosis, symptomatic treatment is sufficient, loperamide to decrease intestinal activity and fluid and electrolyte replacement. Antibiotic treatment is reserved for exceptional cases [91, 94].

Macrophages or mononuclear phagocytes are cells of the immune system, derived from blood monocytes that migrate to tissues where they differentiate into mature macrophages that can live for years. Their main function is phagocytosis of pathogens and cellular debris, although they also participate in inflammatory processes by chemotaxis of other cells of the immune system. They are antigen-presenting cells (APCs) and possess an extraordinary cytokine-producing capacity (TNF-α, IL-1, IL-6, IL-12, etc.) in response to pathogen-associated molecular patterns (PAMPs) [95].

Hui WW et al. studied the ability of infected macrophages to trigger immune responses and thus "alert" inactivated macrophages. This communication is carried out by exosomes; this allows macrophages to perform their function and, in addition, due to the possession of lipopolysaccharides by the exosomes, causes an inflammatory reaction to be exerted [39].

Years later, this researcher and his group, due to the lack of an approved vaccine for humans, delved deeper into macrophage exosomes. They studied the proteome of the exosomes of Salmonella-infected macrophages. They observed that, once the exosomes are administered, the body's innate and adaptive response is triggered, leading to a release of the aforementioned cytokines and an increase in the production of IgG antibodies. Likewise, when exosomes are administered intranasally, mucosal defences are activated [40].

3.8 *Mycobacterium tuberculosis*

The genus *Mycobacterium* is characterised by aerobic, non-sporulating, non-motile bacilli. The most important bacteria in this group are *Mycobacterium tuberculosis* and *M. bovis*, the aetiological agents of tuberculosis, and *M. leprae*, the aetiological agent of leprosy [96].

Many of the special characteristics of TB bacteria are due to their cell wall chemistry. It has a murein coat, numerous lipids such as glycolipids (cord factor being trehalose dimycolate), mycolic acids, mucosides, and waxes [97].

Primary TB infection is localised in the lungs. In most cases, pathogens enter the lung via respiratory droplets (airborne transmission), where they are phagocytosed by alveolar macrophages (facultative intracellular pathogen). Bacteria are able to reproduce in macrophages due to their ability to inhibit phagolysosome formation (prevents fusion of the phagosome with lysosomes). In about 10% of cases, the primary infection can reactivate in immunocompromised individuals and progress after months or years to a secondary stage characterised by tissue necrosis [98].

TB is an endemic disease. Although it is much less common in developed countries, from a global perspective it remains a priority medical problem. The major reservoir is the human (except for *M. bovis*). The main source of infection is the human carrier; there are no healthy carriers. Transmission of the disease is usually direct, via respiratory droplets [98, 99].

An attenuated vaccine is available that reduces the risk of infection by 5% and contains Bacillus Calmette-Guerin (BCG), which is an attenuated strain of *M. bovis*. Vaccination provides temporary immunity, for a period of 5–10 years. In persons at risk of developing the disease who are: contact tuberculin-positive, immunocompromised tuberculin-positive, or radiologically confirmed residual tuberculosis, isoniazid prophylaxis for 6 months is recommended [98, 99].

The exosomes shed by the cells into the medium, which allows intercellular communication, can be used as potent immunotherapeutic agents to tackle TB. First, it is possible to add immune cell exosomes to the current vaccine against *Mycobacterium tuberculosis* to enhance the immune response and thus make the defence against subsequent infections effective. This possibility as an adjuvant has been tested in hepatitis and has given good results [41]. And secondly, the ability of exosomes to harbour molecules inside them in order to administer the desired drugs, which are unable to cross biological membranes on their own [42].

In the study conducted by Cheng and Schorey, the main objective was to evaluate the therapeutic capabilities of macrophage-derived exosomes in mice infected with tuberculosis bacteria. The researchers were confronted with the fact that, for the vaccine that exists, the protective efficacy decreases over time and the lungs are exposed to the infection. They concluded that both exosomes applied as vaccines, as a booster with the currently available vaccine, exert an immune response via Th1 and Th2, although the latter is more limited. Finally, an increase in IFN-γ and IL-2 levels in lung cells after vaccination was determined by ELISA [43].

3.9 *Toxoplasma gondii*

It is an obligate intracellular parasite that causes toxoplasmosis. It has several life forms:

Tachyzoites: the result of asexual multiplication by endopolygeny or multiple fusion. They are arranged in clusters or pseudocysts. They characterise the acute phase of infection in which rapid multiplication of the parasite occurs [100].

Bradyzoites: asexual reproductive forms formed by endodiogeny or binary fission. They group together to form spherical tissue cysts. They constitute the chronic (latent) phase of infection [100].

Oocysts: form after sexual multiplication in cells of the host (cat) intestinal epithelium. They are excreted in the faeces and to be infective they need to continue sporulation outdoors, which, depending on external conditions, will occur between two and 21 days. In a warm, humid climate, oocysts can persist viable for more than a year [100].

Humans can become infected by ingesting the tissue cysts contained in the meat of infected animals or by ingesting mature oocysts in contaminated food and water. When a woman's primary infection coincides with her pregnancy, the parasite can cross the placental barrier and infect the foetus, resulting in congenital infection [101, 102].

Pyrimethamine, sulphadiazine, and folinic acid are generally used as treatments. In children with congenital toxoplasmosis, pyrimethamine alone is used. In cases of HIV with toxoplasmic encephalitis, if sensitivity to sulphonamides develops, clindamycin is given instead of sulphadiazine. For HIV patients, trimethoprim and sulfamethoxazole (co-trimoxazole) are used as prophylaxis. In pregnant women spiramycin [103–105].

Dendritic cells immunised with *Toxoplasma gondii* producing antigens are effective in coping with the infection and producing an effective immune response. Based on this premise, Aline F and her team developed a vaccine based on exosomes derived from dendritic cells that had been exposed to *T. gondii*. They were able to prove that the response generated is mediated by Th1 lymphocytes. These secrete IL-2 and IFN-gamma, activate macrophages and NK cells. They also promote the function of cytotoxic T-lymphocytes that activate the cell-mediated immune response to intracellular pathogens such as *Toxoplasma gondii* [44].

A woman infected with *T. gondii* is capable of transmitting it to her foetus. In the study by Beauvillain et al., they focus on how the use of exosomes for this pathology can protect the offspring. They tested both parasite-exposed and non-parasite-exposed dendritic cells and exosomes as vaccines. They concluded that, in addition to triggering an effective immune response, it increases fertility, and this is because the immune response is type 2 (Th1-mediated response leads to non-viability of pregnancy due to poor implantation and maintenance of the placenta) [45].

3.10 *Cryptococcus neoformans*

It is a unicellular yeast with a size of 3–5 μm surrounded by a polysaccharide capsule. It inhabits soils rich in organic substances. The most common route of entry in humans is respiratory; organisms are inhaled and reach the lungs. Pulmonary cryptococcosis may develop [106].

From the primary pulmonary focus, pathogens spread via the blood to other organs. *C. neoformans* shows a major affinity for the central nervous system, where it develops very severe meningoencephalitis. The treatment of choice for this disease is amphotericin B and 5-fluorocytosine [106–108].

Oliveira et al. investigated the role of *C. neoformans* exosomes upon entry into the organism. They were able to prove in vitro that these vesicles play a modulating role in infection and the generation of the immune response. The complement system is activated, leading to inflammation, phagocytosis, and cell lysis. Furthermore, when exosomes come into contact with macrophages, they release antimicrobial compounds such as TGF, TNF, and IL-10 [46].

Due to the lack of knowledge about fungal exosomes, they wanted to study them in-depth. They used advanced techniques such as cryogenic electron microscopy and tomography, proteomics (random access liquid chromatography in tandem with mass spectrometry), and nanoscale flow cytometry. They were able to conclude that exosomes can function as stand-alone vaccines and elicit an immune response to confront the pathogen [47].

4. Conclusions and future perspective

Exosome therapies are a major breakthrough in preventive and therapeutic medicine. There are currently 259 ongoing studies involving exosomes according to the clinical trials website ClinicalTrials.gov. In this review, exosomes derived from different cell types are proposed as a therapy for zoonotic infections. The rationale for the use of exosomes, the benefits involved and the fact that MSCs are not used have been outlined above. Due to their immunomodulatory capacity, exosomes will help the immune system to cope with pathologies. They can also be used as vehicles by introducing the desired molecules inside them due to their permeability to biological barriers.

Delivering exosomes intranasally provides faster action, allows smaller doses to achieve the same effect as injection therapy, is non-invasive, avoids the pain typically associated with parenteral therapy, and the potential for side effects is minimal.

Since exosomes trigger the immune system's defence against a variety of zoonotic diseases, further development of their use as vaccines would be important for clinical trials. If finally viable, one option to consider is the creation of a bank of exosomes so that they can be available for both prevention and disease control.

Finally, one option to study would be the possibility that exosomes could fight not just one disease but a spectrum of diseases by activating the immune system and thus boosting the body's defenses. This would make it a universal tool for tackling different pathologies.

Acknowledgements

We want to thank Ramón Wahl for his contribution to the performance of figure and table.

Conflict of interest

The authors declare no conflict of interest.

Author details

Fernando Ojeda[1,2], Gabriela Barreto[2] and Sinforiano J. Posadas[1,2]*

1 Instituto Biotecnológico en Medicina Integrativa y Terapias Avanzadas (INBIOMITER), Promalaga I+D, Malaga, Spain

2 DIBIOTHER ORGANIZACION, Promalaga I+D, Malaga, Spain

*Address all correspondence to: sposman@uma.es

References

[1] Shin B, Park W. Zoonotic diseases and phytochemical medicines for microbial infections in veterinary science: Current state and future perspective. Frontiers in Veterinary Science. 2018;**5**:166. DOI: 10.3389/fvets.2018.00166

[2] Golchin A, Farahany TZ. Biological products: Cellular therapy and FDA approved products. Stem Cell Reviews and Reports. 2019;**15**:166-175. DOI: 10.1007/s12015-018-9866-1

[3] Bruno S, Deregibus MC, Camussi G. The secretome of mesenchymal stromal cells: Role of extracellular vesicles in immunomodulation. Immunology Letters. 2015;**168**:154-158. DOI: 10.1016/j.imlet.2015.06.007

[4] Di Rocco G, Baldari S, Toietta G. Towards therapeutic delivery of extracellular vesicles: Strategies for in vivo tracking and biodistribution analysis. Stem Cells International. 2016;**2016**:1-12. DOI: 10.1155/2016/5029619

[5] Ludwig AK, Giebel B. Exosomes: Small vesicles participating in intercellular communication. The International Journal of Biochemistry & Cell Biology. 2012;**44**:11-15. DOI: 10.1016/j.biocel.2011.10.005

[6] Rani S, Ryan AE, Griffin MD, Ritter T. Mesenchymal stem cell-derived extracellular vesicles: Toward cell-free therapeutic applications. Molecular Therapy. 2015;**23**:812-823. DOI: 10.1038/mt.2015.44

[7] van der Pol E, Böing AN, Harrison P, Sturk A, Nieuwland R. Classification, functions, and clinical relevance of extracellular vesicles. Pharmacological Reviews. 2012;**64**:676-705. DOI: 10.1124/pr.112.005983

[8] Février B, Raposo G. Exosomes: Endosomal-derived vesicles shipping extracellular messages. Current Opinion in Cell Biology. 2004;**16**:415-421. DOI: 10.1016/j.ceb.2004.06.003

[9] Pan BT, Teng K, Wu C, Adam M, Johnstone RM. Electron microscopic evidence for externalization of the transferrin receptor in vesicular form in sheep reticulocytes. The Journal of Cell Biology. 1985;**101**:942-948. DOI: 10.1083/jcb.101.3.942

[10] Natasha G, Gundogan B, Tan A, et al. Exosomes as immunotheranostic nanoparticles. Clinical Therapeutics. 2014;**36**:820-829. DOI: 10.1016/j.clinthera.2014.04.019

[11] Kalinina N, Kharlampieva D, Loguinova M, et al. Characterization of secretomes provides evidence for adipose-derived mesenchymal stromal cells subtypes. Stem Cell Research & Therapy. 2015;**6**:1-12. DOI: 10.1186/s13287-015-0209-8

[12] Zhu X, Badawi M, Pomeroy S, et al. Comprehensive toxicity and immunogenicity studies reveal minimal effects in mice following sustained dosing of extracellular vesicles derived from HEK293T cells. Journal of Extracellular Vesicles. 2017;**6**:1-11. DOI: 10.1080/20013078.2017.1324730

[13] Bari E, Ferrarotti I, Torre ML, Corsico AG, Perteghella S. Mesenchymal stem/stromal cell secretome for lung regeneration: The long way through "pharmaceuticalization" for the best formulation. Journal of Controlled

Release. 2019;**309**:11-24. DOI: 10.1016/j.jconrel.2019.07.022

[14] Tran TH, Mattheolabakis G, Aldawsari H, Amiji M. Exosomes as nanocarriers for immunotherapy of cancer and inflammatory diseases. Clinical Immunology. 2015;**160**:46-58. DOI: 10.1016/j.clim.2015.03.021

[15] De Jong OG, Van Balkom BW, Schiffelers RM, Bouten CV, Verhaar MC. Extracellular vesicles: Potential roles in regenerative medicine. Frontiers in Immunology. 2014;**5**:1-13. DOI: 10.3389/fimmu.2014.00608

[16] Wang J, Wu F, Liu C, et al. Exosomes released from rabies virus-infected cells may be involved in the infection process. Virologica Sinica. 2019;**34**:59-65. DOI: 10.1007/s12250-019-00087-3

[17] Yang J, Zhang X, Chen X, Wang L, Yang G. Exosome mediated delivery of miR-124 promotes neurogenesis after ischemia. Molecular Therapy Nucleic Acids. 2017;7:278-287. DOI: 10.1016/j.omtn.2017.04.010

[18] Alvarez-Erviti L, Seow Y, Yin H, Betts C, Lakhal S, Wood MJ. Delivery of siRNA to the mouse brain by systemic injection of targeted exosomes. Nature Biotechnology. 2011;**29**:341-345. DOI: 10.1038/nbt.1807

[19] Kumar P, Wu H, McBride JL, et al. Transvascular delivery of small interfering RNA to the central nervous system. Nature. 2007;**448**:39-43. DOI: 10.1038/nature05901

[20] Wang J, Teng Y, Zhao G, et al. Exosome-mediated delivery of inducible miR-423-5p enhances resistance of MRC-5 cells to rabies virus infection. International Journal of Molecular Sciences. 2019;**20**:1-15. DOI: 10.3390/ijms20071537

[21] Pleet ML, Erickson J, DeMarino C, et al. Ebola virus VP40 modulates cell cycle and biogenesis of extracellular vesicles. The Journal of Infectious Diseases. 2018;**218**:365-387. DOI: 10.1093/infdis/jiy472

[22] Record M, Subra C, Silvente-Poirot S, Poirot M. Exosomes as intercellular signalosomes and pharmacological effectors. Biochemical Pharmacology. 2011;**81**:1171-1182. DOI: 10.1016/j.bcp.2011.02.011

[23] Anticoli S, Manfredi F, Chiozzini C, et al. An exosome-based vaccine platform imparts cytotoxic T lymphocyte immunity against viral antigens. Biotechnology Journal. 2018;**13**:1-18. DOI: 10.1002/biot.201700443

[24] Shrivastava S, Ray RM, Holguin L, et al. Exosome-mediated stable epigenetic repression of HIV-1. Nature Communications. 2021;**12**:1-14. DOI: 10.1038/s41467-021-25839-2

[25] Tang X, Lu H, Dooner M, Chapman S, Quesenberry PJ, Ramratnam B. Exosomal tat protein activates latent HIV-1 in primary, resting CD4+ T lymphocytes. JCI Insight. 2018;**3**:1-14. DOI: 10.1172/jci.insight.95676

[26] Cruz FF, Rocco PRM. Stem-cell extracellular vesicles and lung repair. Stem Cell Investigation. 2017;**4**:1-11. DOI: 10.21037/sci.2017.09.02

[27] Abraham A, Krasnodembskaya A. Mesenchymal stem cell-derived extracellular vesicles for the treatment of acute respiratory distress syndrome. Stem Cells Translational Medicine. 2020;**9**:28-38. DOI: 10.1002/sctm.19-0205

[28] Tang XD, Shi L, Monsel A, et al. Mesenchymal stem cell microvesicles attenuate acute lung injury in mice

partly mediated by Ang-1 mRNA. Stem Cells. 2017;**35**:1849-1859. DOI: 10.1002/stem.2619

[29] Jiang L, Driedonks TAP, Jong WSP, et al. A bacterial extracellular vesicle-based intranasal vaccine against SARS-CoV-2 protects against disease and elicits neutralizing antibodies to wild-type and Delta variants. Journal of Extracellular Vesicles. 2022;**11**:1-34. DOI: 10.1002/jev2.12192

[30] Frank-Cannon TC, Alto LT, McAlpine FE, Tansey MG. Does neuroinflammation fan the flame in neurodegenerative diseases? Molecular Neurodegeneration. 2009;**4**:1-13. DOI: 10.1186/1750-1326-4-47

[31] Serrano-Castro PJ, Estivill-Torrús G, Cabezudo-García P, et al. Impact of SARS-CoV-2 infection on neurodegenerative and neuropsychiatric diseases: a delayed pandemic?. Influencia de la infección SARS-CoV-2 sobre enfermedades neurodegenerativas y neuropsiquiátricas: ¿una pandemia demorada? Neurología (English Edition). 2020;**35**:245-251. DOI: 10.1016/j.nrl.2020.04.002

[32] Baig AM, Khaleeq A, Ali U, Syeda H. Evidence of the COVID-19 virus targeting the CNS: Tissue distribution, host-virus interaction, and proposed neurotropic mechanisms. ACS Chemical Neuroscience. 2020;**11**:995-998. DOI: 10.1021/acschemneuro.0c00122

[33] Liu YM, Tseng CH, Chen YC, et al. Exosome-delivered and Y RNA-derived small RNA suppresses influenza virus replication. Journal of Biomedical Science. 2019;**26**:1-14. DOI: 10.1186/s12929-019-0553-6

[34] Maemura T, Fukuyama S, Sugita Y, et al. Lung-derived Exosomal miR-483-3p regulates the innate immune response to influenza virus infection. The Journal of Infectious Diseases. 2018;**217**:1372-1382. DOI: 10.1093/infdis/jiy035

[35] Loy H, Kuok DIT, Hui KPY, et al. Therapeutic implications of human umbilical cord mesenchymal stromal cells in attenuating influenza a(H5N1) virus-associated acute lung injury. The Journal of Infectious Diseases. 2019;**219**:186-196. DOI: 10.1093/infdis/jiy478

[36] Yi J, Wang Y, Zhang H, et al. Interferon-inducible transmembrane protein 3-containing exosome as a new carrier for the cell-to-cell transmission of anti-Brucella activity. Frontiers in Veterinary Science. 2021;**8**:1-11. DOI: 10.3389/fvets.2021.642968

[37] Wellington D, Laurenson-Schafer H, Abdel-Haq A, Dong T. IFITM3: How genetics influence influenza infection demographically. Biomedical Journal. 2019;**42**:19-26. DOI: 10.1016/j.bj.2019.01.004

[38] Solanki KS, Varshney R, Qureshi S, et al. Non-infectious outer membrane vesicles derived from Brucella abortus S19Δper as an alternative acellular vaccine protects mice against virulent challenge. International Immunopharmacology. 2021;**90**:1-14. DOI: 10.1016/j.intimp.2020.107148

[39] Hui WW, Hercik K, Belsare S, et al. Salmonella enterica Serovar typhimurium alters the extracellular proteome of macrophages and leads to the production of proinflammatory exosomes. Infection and Immunity. 2018;**86**:1-21. DOI: 10.1128/IAI.00386-17

[40] Hui WW, Emerson LE, Clapp B, et al. Antigen-encapsulating host extracellular vesicles derived from Salmonella-infected cells stimulate

pathogen-specific Th1-type responses in vivo. PLoS Pathogens. 2021;**17**:1-27. DOI: 10.1371/journal.ppat.1009465

[41] Jesus S, Soares E, Cruz MT, Borges O. Exosomes as adjuvants for the recombinant hepatitis B antigen: First report. European Journal of Pharmaceutics and Biopharmaceutics. 2018;**133**:1-11. DOI: 10.1016/j.ejpb.2018.09.029

[42] Das CK, Jena BC, Banerjee I, Das S, Parekh A, Bhutia SK, et al. Exosome as a novel shuttle for delivery of therapeutics across biological barriers. Molecular Pharmaceutics. 2019;**16**:24-40. DOI: 10.1021/acs.molpharmaceut.8b00901

[43] Cheng Y, Schorey JS. Exosomes carrying mycobacterial antigens can protect mice against mycobacterium tuberculosis infection. European Journal of Immunology. 2013;**43**:3279-3290. DOI: 10.1002/eji.201343727

[44] Aline F, Bout D, Amigorena S, Roingeard P, Dimier-Poisson I. Toxoplasma gondii antigen-pulsed-dendritic cell-derived exosomes induce a protective immune response against T. gondii infection. Infection and Immunity. 2004;**72**:4127-4137. DOI: 10.1128/IAI.72.7.4127-4137.2004

[45] Beauvillain C, Juste MO, Dion S, Pierre J, Dimier-Poisson I. Exosomes are an effective vaccine against congenital toxoplasmosis in mice. Vaccine. 2009;**27**:1750-1757. DOI: 10.1016/j.vaccine.2009.01.022

[46] Oliveira DL, Freire-de-Lima CG, Nosanchuk JD, Casadevall A, Rodrigues ML, Nimrichter L. Extracellular vesicles from *Cryptococcus neoformans* modulate macrophage functions. Infection and Immunity. 2010;**78**:1601-1609. DOI: 10.1128/IAI.01171-09

[47] Rizzo J, Wong SSW, Gazi AD, et al. Cryptococcus extracellular vesicles properties and their use as vaccine platforms. Journal of Extracellular Vesicles. 2021;**10**:1-19. DOI: 10.1002/jev2.12129

[48] Rabia [Internet]. Organización Mundial de la Salud. 2020. Available from: https://www.who.int/es/news-room/fact-sheets/detail/rabies [Accessed 2022-03-14]

[49] Tordo N, Poch O, Ermine A, Keith G, Rougeon F. Walking along the rabies genome: Is the large G-L intergenic region a remnant gene? Proceedings of the National Academy of Sciences of the United States of America. 1986;**83**: 3914-3918. DOI: 10.1073/pnas.83.11.3914

[50] Hicks DJ, Fooks AR, Johnson N. Developments in rabies vaccines. Clinical and Experimental Immunology. 2012;**169**:199-204. DOI: 10.1111/j.1365-2249.2012.04592.x

[51] Armbruster N, Jasny E, Petsch B. Advances in RNA vaccines for preventive indications: A case study of a vaccine against rabies. Vaccines (Basel). 2019;**7**:132. DOI: 10.3390/vaccines7040132

[52] Warrell MJ, Warrell DA. Rabies and other lyssavirus diseases. Lancet. 2004;**363**:959-969. DOI: 10.1016/S0140-6736(04)15792-9

[53] Alenquer M, Amorim MJ. Exosome biogenesis, regulation, and function in viral infection. Viruses. 2015;**7**:5066-5083. DOI: 10.3390/v7092862

[54] Simons M, Raposo G. Exosomes—Vesicular carriers for intercellular communication. Current Opinion in Cell Biology. 2009;**21**:575-581. DOI: 10.1016/j.ceb.2009.03.007

[55] Jacob ST, Crozier I, Fischer WA 2nd, et al. Ebola virus disease. Nature Reviews. Disease Primers. 2020;**6**:1-31. DOI: 10.1038/s41572-020-0147-3

[56] Enfermedad por el virus del Ébola. Organización Mundial de la Salud [Internet]. 2021. Available from: https://www.who.int/es/news-room/fact-sheets/detail/ebola-virus-disease [Accessed: March 17, 2022]

[57] Schmidt ME, Varga SM. The CD8 T cell response to respiratory virus infections. Frontiers in Immunology. 2018;**9**:1-12. DOI: 10.3389/fimmu.2018.00678

[58] McElroy AK, Akondy RS, Davis CW, et al. Human Ebola virus infection results in substantial immune activation. Proceedings of the National Academy of Sciences of the United States of America. 2015;**112**:4719-4724. DOI: 10.1073/pnas.1502619112

[59] Sullivan NJ, Hensley L, Asiedu C, et al. CD8+ cellular immunity mediates rAd5 vaccine protection against Ebola virus infection of nonhuman primates. Nature Medicine. 2011;**17**:1128-1131. DOI: 10.1038/nm.2447

[60] Schorey JS, Cheng Y, Singh PP, Smith VL. Exosomes and other extracellular vesicles in host-pathogen interactions. EMBO Reports. 2015;**16**:24-43. DOI: 10.15252/embr.201439363

[61] Mathivanan S, Ji H, Simpson RJ. Exosomes: Extracellular organelles important in intercellular communication. Journal of Proteomics. 2010;**73**:1907-1920. DOI: 10.1016/j.jprot.2010.06.006

[62] Fanales-Belasio E, Raimondo M, Suligoi B, Buttò S. HIV virology and pathogenetic mechanisms of infection: A brief overview. Annali dell'Istituto Superiore di Sanità. 2010;**46**:5-14. DOI: 10.4415/ANN_10_01_02

[63] Melikyan GB. HIV entry: A game of hide-and-fuse? Current Opinion in Virology. 2014;**4**:1-7. DOI: 10.1016/j.coviro.2013.09.004

[64] Simon V, Ho DD, Abdool KQ. HIV/AIDS epidemiology, pathogenesis, prevention, and treatment. Lancet. 2006;**368**:489-504. DOI: 10.1016/S0140-6736(06)69157-5

[65] VIH/sida. Organización Mundial de la Salud [Internet]. 2021. Available from: https://www.who.int/es/news-room/fact-sheets/detail/hiv-aids [Accessed: March 19, 2022]

[66] Mahajan SD, Ordain NS, Kutscher H, Karki S, Reynolds JL. HIV neuroinflammation: The role of exosomes in cell signaling, prognostic and diagnostic biomarkers and drug delivery. Frontiers in Cell and Development Biology. 2021;**9**:1-9. DOI: 10.3389/fcell.2021.637192

[67] Cui J, Li F, Shi ZL. Origin and evolution of pathogenic coronaviruses. Nature Reviews. Microbiology. 2019;**17**:181-192. DOI: 10.1038/s41579-018-0118-9

[68] Su S, Wong G, Shi W, et al. Epidemiology, genetic recombination, and pathogenesis of coronaviruses. Trends in Microbiology. 2016;**24**:490-502. DOI: 10.1016/j.tim.2016.03.003

[69] Yu F, Du L, Ojcius DM, Pan C, Jiang S. Measures for diagnosing and treating infections by a novel coronavirus responsible for a pneumonia outbreak originating in Wuhan, China. Microbes and Infection. 2020;**22**:74-79. DOI: 10.1016/j.micinf.2020.01.003

[70] Guan Y, Zheng BJ, He YQ, et al. Isolation and characterization of viruses

related to the SARS coronavirus from animals in southern China. Science. 2003;**302**:276-278. DOI: 10.1126/science.1087139

[71] Hemida MG, Perera RA, Wang P, et al. Middle East respiratory syndrome (MERS) coronavirus seroprevalence in domestic livestock in Saudi Arabia, 2010 to 2013. Euro Surveillance. 2013;**18**:20659. DOI: 10.2807/1560-7917.es2013.18.50.20659

[72] Qiang XL, Xu P, Fang G, Liu WB, Kou Z. Using the spike protein feature to predict infection risk and monitor the evolutionary dynamic of coronavirus. Infectious Diseases of Poverty. 2020;**9**:1-8. DOI: 10.1186/s40249-020-00649-8

[73] Mackenzie JS, Childs JE, Field HE, Wang LF, Breed AC. The role of bats as reservoir hosts of emerging neuroviruses. Neurotropic Viral Infections. 2016;**2**:403-454. DOI: 10.1007/978-3-319-33189-8_12

[74] Hamming I, Timens W, Bulthuis ML, Lely AT, Navis G, van Goor H. Tissue distribution of ACE2 protein, the functional receptor for SARS coronavirus. A first step in understanding SARS pathogenesis. The Journal of Pathology. 2004;**203**:631-637. DOI: 10.1002/path.1570

[75] Belouzard S, Millet JK, Licitra BN, Whittaker GR. Mechanisms of coronavirus cell entry mediated by the viral spike protein. Viruses. 2012;**4**:1011-1033. DOI: 10.3390/v4061011

[76] Zhu N, Zhang D, Wang W, et al. A novel coronavirus from patients with pneumonia in China, 2019. The New England Journal of Medicine. 2020;**382**:727-733. DOI: 10.1056/NEJMoa2001017

[77] Li Q, Guan X, Wu P, et al. Early transmission dynamics in Wuhan, China, of novel coronavirus-infected pneumonia. The New England Journal of Medicine. 2020;**382**:1199-1207. DOI: 10.1056/NEJMoa2001316

[78] Wu Z, McGoogan JM. Characteristics of and important lessons from the coronavirus disease 2019 (COVID-19) outbreak in China: Summary of a report of 72 314 cases from the Chinese Center for Disease Control and Prevention. Journal of the American Medical Association. 2020;**323**:1239-1242. DOI: 10.1001/jama.2020.2648

[79] Ministerio de Sanidad [Internet]. 2021. Available from: https://www.sanidad.gob.es/ [Accessed: March 25, 2022]

[80] Vacunas contra la COVID-19. Organización Mundial de la Salud [Internet]. 2021. Available from: https://www.who.int/es/emergencies/diseases/novel-coronavirus-2019/covid-19-vaccines [Accessed: March 28, 2022]

[81] Virus de la gripe aviar y otros virus de la gripe de origen zoonótico. Organización Mundial de la Salud [Internet]. 2018. Available from: https://www.who.int/es/news-room/fact-sheets/detail/influenza-(avian-and-other-zoonotic) [Accessed: March 27, 2022]

[82] De Vlugt C, Sikora D, Pelchat M. Insight into influenza: A virus cap-snatching. Viruses. 2018;**10**:1-7. DOI: 10.3390/v10110641

[83] Luo M. Influenza virus entry. Advances in Experimental Medicine and Biology. 2012;**726**:201-221. DOI: 10.1007/978-1-4614-0980-9_9

[84] Arcanjo AC, Mazzocco G, de Oliveira SF, Plewczynski D, Radomski JP. Role of the host genetic variability in the influenza A virus susceptibility. Acta Biochimica Polonica. 2014;**61**:403-419. DOI: 10.18388/ABP.2014_1858

[85] Kim H, Webster RG, Webby RJ. Influenza virus: Dealing with a drifting and shifting pathogen. Viral Immunology. 2018;**31**:174-183. DOI: 10.1089/vim.2017.0141

[86] González-Espinoza G, Arce-Gorvel V, Mémet S, Gorvel JP. Brucella: Reservoirs and niches in animals and humans. Pathogens. 2021;**10**:1-21. DOI: 10.3390/pathogens10020186

[87] Brucelosis. Organización Mundial de la Salud [Internet]. 2020. Available from: https://www.who.int/es/news-room/fact-sheets/detail/brucellosis [Accessed: March 29, 2022]

[88] Głowacka P, Żakowska D, Naylor K, Niemcewicz M, Bielawska-Drózd A. Brucella—Virulence factors, pathogenesis and treatment. Polish Journal of Microbiology. 2018;**67**:151-161. DOI: 10.21307/pjm-2018-029

[89] Fiebre tifoidea. Organización Mundial de la Salud [Internet]. 2018. Available from: https://www.who.int/es/news-room/fact-sheets/detail/typhoid [Accessed: March 30, 2022]

[90] Spanò S. Mechanisms of *Salmonella typhi* host restriction. Advances in Experimental Medicine and Biology. 2016;**915**:283-294. DOI: 10.1007/978-3-319-32189-9_17

[91] Salmonella (no tifoidea). Organización Mundial de la Salud [Internet]. 2018. Available from: https://www.who.int/es/news-room/fact-sheets/detail/salmonella-(non-typhoidal) [Accessed: March 27, 2022]

[92] Andino A, Hanning I. *Salmonella enterica*: Survival, colonization, and virulence differences among serovars. ScientificWorldJournal. 2015;**2015**:1-16. DOI: 10.1155/2015/520179

[93] Zhang CZ, Zhang Y, Ding XM, et al. Emergence of ciprofloxacin heteroresistance in foodborne *Salmonella enterica* serovar Agona. The Journal of Antimicrobial Chemotherapy. 2020;**75**:2773-2779. DOI: 10.1093/jac/dkaa288

[94] Lääveri T, Sterne J, Rombo L, Kantele A. Systematic review of loperamide: No proof of antibiotics being superior to loperamide in treatment of mild/moderate travellers' diarrhoea. Travel Medicine and Infectious Disease. 2016;**14**:299-312. DOI: 10.1016/j.tmaid.2016.06.006

[95] Shapouri-Moghaddam A, Mohammadian S, Vazini H, et al. Macrophage plasticity, polarization, and function in health and disease. Journal of Cellular Physiology. 2018;**233**:6425-6440. DOI: 10.1002/jcp.26429

[96] Bañuls AL, Sanou A, Van Anh NT, Godreuil S. Mycobacterium tuberculosis: Ecology and evolution of a human bacterium. Journal of Medical Microbiology. 2015;**64**:1261-1269. DOI: 10.1099/jmm.0.000171

[97] Brennan PJ. Structure, function, and biogenesis of the cell wall of *Mycobacterium tuberculosis*. Tuberculosis (Edinburgh, Scotland). 2003;**83**:91-97. DOI: 10.1016/s1472-9792(02)00089-6

[98] Tuberculosis. Organización Mundial de la Salud [Internet]. 2021. Available from: https://www.who.int/es/news-room/fact-sheets/detail/tuberculosis [Accessed: March 28, 2022]

[99] Suárez I, Fünger SM, Kröger S, Rademacher J, Fätkenheuer G, Rybniker J. The diagnosis and treatment of tuberculosis. Deutsches Ärzteblatt International. 2019;**116**:729-735. DOI: 10.3238/arztebl.2019.0729

[100] Lourido S. *Toxoplasma gondii*. Trends in Parasitology. 2019;**35**:944-945. DOI: 10.1016/j.pt.2019.07.001

[101] Zhao XY, Ewald SE. The molecular biology and immune control of chronic *Toxoplasma gondii* infection. The Journal of Clinical Investigation. 2020;**130**:3370-3380. DOI: 10.1172/JCI136226

[102] Marra CM. Central nervous system infection with *Toxoplasma gondii*. Handbook of Clinical Neurology. 2018;**152**:117-122. DOI: 10.1016/B978-0-444-63849-6.00009-8

[103] de-la-Torre A, Gómez-Marín J. Disease of the year 2019: ocular toxoplasmosis in HIV-infected patients. Ocular Immunology & Inflammation. 2020;**28**:1031-1039. DOI: 10.1080/09273948.2020.1735450

[104] Jafarpour Azami S, Mohammad Rahimi H, Mirjalali H, Zali MR. Unravelling toxoplasma treatment: Conventional drugs toward nanomedicine. World Journal of Microbiology and Biotechnology. 2021;**37**:1-9. DOI: 10.1007/s11274-021-03000-x

[105] Furtado JM, Smith JR, Belfort R Jr, Gattey D, Winthrop KL. Toxoplasmosis: A global threat. Journal of Global Infectious Diseases. 2011;**3**:281-284. DOI: 10.4103/0974-777X.83536

[106] Srikanta D, Santiago-Tirado FH, Doering TL. Cryptococcus neoformans: Historical curiosity to modern pathogen. Yeast. 2014;**31**:47-60. DOI: 10.1002/yea.2997

[107] Alspaugh JA. Virulence mechanisms and *Cryptococcus neoformans* pathogenesis. Fungal Genetics and Biology. 2015;**78**:55-58. DOI: 10.1016/j.fgb.2014.09.004

[108] Brilhante RSN, Rocha MGD, Oliveira JS, et al. *Cryptococcus neoformans*/*Cryptococcus gattii* species complex melanized by epinephrine: Increased yeast survival after amphotericin B exposure. Microbial Pathogenesis. 2020;**143**:1-19. DOI: 10.1016/j.micpath.2020.104123

Chapter 8

Emerging and Re-Emerging Bacterial Zoonoses: A Nigerian Perspective on Control, Prevention and Intervention

Andrew W. Taylor-Robinson and Olaitan O. Omitola

Abstract

A propensity to re-emerge is a characteristic of bacterial zoonoses, diseases caused by bacteria that can be transmitted to humans from animals. Research shows that their transmission occurs in Nigeria, the most populated nation in Africa. However, due to insufficient epidemiological surveillance of bacterial zoonoses, the magnitude and burden of these infectious diseases is not fully acknowledged. They are therefore not a priority target of the national public health policy. This lesser concern is regardless of their likely role in the extensive prevalence of non-malarial undifferentiated fever in Nigeria. Several animal reservoirs and arthropod vectors of transmission have been identified for these diseases, Yet, the increase in cases of undiagnosed febrile illness emphasizes the imperative to undertake an extensive evaluation of other possible reservoirs, vectors and transmission cycles that may raise the local risk of zoonotic bacterial infections. Animal health interventions have been advanced as an economically viable and practical approach. Further, facilitating the operation of a community-based One Health program is essential to providing the comprehensive epidemiological information that is required in order to improve prioritization of bacterial zoonoses. This would generate impetus for much-needed investment in relevant public health interventions.

Keywords: bacterium, emerging, zoonosis, vector, reservoir, transmission, infectious disease, fever, public health, Nigeria, One Health

1. Introduction

Diseases that are transmitted directly or indirectly from wildlife to humans are a major cause of morbidity and mortality globally, including in Nigeria, which has the largest population and economy in Africa [1]. Around 60% of the 1500 or more infectious microorganisms known to be human pathogens are recognized as zoonotic, i.e. they normally exist in animals but they can also infect humans [2, 3]. While approximately 73% of emerging and re-emerging pathogens cause zoonotic diseases [2, 3], even more prevalent infectious diseases of major public health importance worldwide, notably malaria and HIV/AIDS, are known to be of zoonotic origin [2]. It is therefore speculated that future generations may face a higher risk of exposure to zoonotic diseases, requiring us to acknowledge the potential impact of this on life expectancy and quality of health [2, 3].

Zoonotic bacterial diseases such as bubonic plague and bovine tuberculosis inflicted enormous damage on mankind during the medieval period, an age in which sanitary measures, vaccines and antibiotics did not exist. In this context, the increasing occurrence and spread of zoonotic bacteria is of concern worldwide, with animals frequently identified as the reservoir host of a wide variety of potential pathogens [3]. The livelihoods of more than 600 million people globally are thought to depend directly on livestock. These communities represent 70% of the poor and marginalized population who are most at risk of zoonotic diseases but are often isolated from adequate health care provision [4].

Bacterial zoonoses are a category of much neglected human infections that may account for a substantial proportion of febrile illnesses without focal features, especially in malaria-endemic hotspots of sub-Saharan Africa, where they are often misdiagnosed as the more familiar protozoan infection [5]. While there are no reported estimates of the prevalence of fever of unknown origin (FUO) in Nigeria records suggest both its common occurrence and incorrect determination of the etiology [6, 7]. Despite the incidence of FUO and although humans have obvious contact with animal reservoirs and vectors of zoonotic disease, potentially important pyrogenic pathogens have not been rigorously investigated in many low- and middle-income countries, particularly in rural areas [8]. A deeper knowledge of the preventable and treatable infectious causes of severe febrile illness is critical to achieving a high level of disease control in developing countries and improving outcomes of affected patients [8].

This chapter discusses the neglected zoonotic bacterial pathogens of Nigeria, West Africa [9]. The focus is on commonly occurring emerging and re-emerging zoonotic diseases, presenting key developments in the field from recent worldwide research, highlighting findings from Nigerian investigations to date and identifying pivotal epidemiological features that have not been described in local studies. Adopting the One Health concept to combat bacterial zoonoses in Nigeria invokes a collaborative, interdisciplinary and multi-sectorial strategy to human and animal health management and interventions. The knowledge gleaned from implementing these principles can be applied in similar West African settings as well as low-income contexts elsewhere.

2. Bacterial zoonoses of public health relevance to Nigeria

As they are frequently associated with high case fatality rates, zoonoses dominate Nigeria's register of notifiable infectious diseases for which emergency declaration is required [10]. Notable zoonotic diseases in Nigeria include Lassa fever, Ebola virus disease, rabies, influenza, yellow fever, anthrax, plague, tuberculosis, salmonellosis and trypanosomiasis, most of which are endemic [1, 10, 11]. Cryptosporidiosis and food-borne *Campylobacter* and *Escherichia coli* O157:H7 infections also constitute important national zoonotic diseases [1]. Leptospirosis, scabies, pentastomiasis and African histoplasmosis occur sporadically [1]. Considered endemic throughout the developing world, neglected zoonoses are inherently capable of causing local outbreaks and larger epidemics [12].

Zoonotic bacterial infections show tremendous potential to re-emerge once they are considered eradicated or under control, and therefore pose grievous, enduring threats to public health [3]. Although re-emerging across sub-Saharan Africa bacterial zoonoses are mostly neglected and under-reported in low-income nations [12]. However, they are acknowledged to be common and widely distributed in Nigeria [13]. Their emergence and re-emergence have been attributed to a combination of climatic, ecological, agricultural and socio-economic factors that create an uncertain public health situation [1].

In a recent investigation, a trend towards disease outbreak in Nigeria was reported for zoonoses of *Leptospira*, a Gram-negative, obligate aerobe spirochete [14]. Leptospirosis is an important bacterial zoonosis, especially in northern Nigeria, with a significant level of sporadic occurrences [1]. A national average incidence of six clinical cases of leptospirosis is reported annually, which is considered to be an underestimate [15]. Research during the past two decades in different regions of Nigeria have detected by serology and urinalysis various serovars of *Leptospira interrogans*, including Canicola and Hardjo, which are considered pathogenic in other continents [14, 16–19].

Possibly the first report of the Gram-negative coccobacillus *Yersinia pseudotuberculosis* in the tropics was from Plateau State, Nigeria, and gastrointestinal yersiniosis due to infection with the pathogenic *Yersinia enterocolitica* is also known [20, 21]. Various serotypes of the Gram-negative, motile bacillus *Campylobacter jejuni* emerged in Nigeria decades ago as prominent causes of human gastroenteritis, inflammation of the stomach and small intestine [1]. Infection due to *C. jejuni* and the other primary zoonotic agent of campylobacteriosis, *Campylobacter coli*, have been on the increase worldwide and often exceed salmonellosis and shigellosis in national notifications [22]. Although comprehensive information on zoonotic campylobacteriosis in Nigeria is limited, both *C. jejuni* and *C. coli* have been isolated [22–24]. Globally, campylobacteriosis and non-typhoidal salmonellosis constitute the most prominent and significant enteric zoonoses [24].

Salmonella enterica serovars Typhimurium and Enteritidis are the main causative agents of sporadic outbreaks of salmonellosis among Africans, with which observations in Ibadan, the capital city of Oyo State, Nigeria, are consistent [25–27]. However, other less common serovars of the Gram-negative, flagellate, facultatively aerobic bacillus have a more geographically restricted distribution. For instance, the rare *S. enterica* Hidudiffy was the predominantly detected serovar in a study in northern Nigeria but was absent in a similar investigation in the southern region [25, 27]. This was attributable to factors like variation in climate or farming systems between the two regions and may need verification [25]. Other rare serovars that have been detected in Nigeria include *S. enterica* Apapa, Mouschaui and Vinohrady [25, 28]. In a recent large-scale surveillance program in Nigeria, *S. enterica* Eko was identified as a major serovar, one of 17 different serotypes that are potentially being transmitted locally within the country [27].

Brucellosis also remains a major neglected zoonotic disease of low-income nations. While assessment of existing data suggests ongoing transmission of human brucellosis in Nigeria, information on the causative *Brucella spp.* Gram-negative, facultative coccobacilli is not sufficiently clear from the limited bacteriological studies [12, 29]. Other common zoonotic bacterial infections, such as bartonellosis, borreliosis, Q fever and rickettsiosis, are also on the rise globally, especially in developing countries like Nigeria [3, 8]. Another Gram-negative coccobacillus, *Coxiella burnetii*, which causes Q fever in humans, has been reported at high serological prevalence in West African countries and has also been detected in veterinary studies in Nigeria [30]. Species of the Gram-negative *Bartonella* such as *B. elizabethae, B. grahamii*, known to cause human diseases in Peru and Thailand [31, 32], were recorded in a Nigerian study [33]. Another investigation identified *Bartonella spp*. in Nigeria similar to those detected in Ghana and Kenya [7]. Several studies have also detected rickettsiae, Gram-negative, intracellular coccobacilli, as potential agents of zoonoses in the country [34, 35]. *Rickettsia massiliae*, *Rickettsia conorii israelensis* and *Rickettsia africae*-like species have been identified as agents of bacterial zoonoses with possible ongoing transmission in Nigeria while *Rickettsia felis*, a prominent emerging rickettsial pathogen that is common in Senegal and Kenya [36], has a largely unknown epidemiology in the rest of the Africa, including Nigeria [30, 34–36].

Together with the isolation of other Gram-negative bacterial zoonotic agents in Nigeria, such as *Anaplasma platys* and *Candidatus Neoehrlichia mikurensis*, its first known description in Africa [34, 35], the scenario presented is of an increasing threat of bacterial zoonotic infections to Nigerian public health. However, fewer studies are conducted to investigate this class of zoonosis than most other infectious agents across a large geographic footprint of the developing world [8]. Plague is an important re-emergent bacterial zoonosis caused by *Yersinia pestis*, one of the most extensively studied pathogenic bacteria. Yet, with current case reports restricted to Africa, there is no known incidence in Nigeria [37, 38]. It is recognized that most zoonotic infections in the country are documented either poorly or not at all, comprehensive efforts to characterize the zoonotic agents are insufficient, and data on important aspects of their epidemiology are also limited [1, 13].

2.1 Infection risks associated with common transmission routes of zoonoses

Close contact with animals due to a person's lifestyle choices or occupation is often associated with the re-emergence and heightened risk of zoonotic bacterial infections. Among others, this subjects farmers, hunters, wildlife workers, veterinarians, pet traders, families with pets, butchers and slaughterhouse workers to an increased risk of transfer of infection from animals [3, 10]. Therefore, bacterial zoonoses are generally considered occupational diseases in Nigeria [10, 14], where intimate proximity to animals as well as exposure to their tissues and body fluids are principal risk factors for zoonotic disease transmission. A prime example is that of leptospirosis during livestock slaughter and processing in abattoirs [14].

Infections with *Brucella* and *Leptospira* have been associated with handling of wild and domestic animals, through which direct transmission may occur [29, 39]. Association with livestock and pets in northern Nigeria increases the risk of *Leptospira* infection acquired through abraded skin when carelessly handling infected animals and their fluids or tissues [14, 15]. However, a significant link between a person's intimate proximity to livestock or other animals and their contracting leptospirosis is not corroborated by inconsistent observations from other countries, thereby suggesting a complexity of region- and context-specific factors in infection risk [40]. Since studies of leptospirosis in Nigeria are limited [40], concentrated in the north and performed on standard risk groups [14, 15], whether such disparity occurs across varied settings in all regions of the country requires further investigation.

Indirect transmission routes for leptospirosis include soil and water contaminated with urine or other body fluids from infected animals via which *L. interrogans* may enter the human body through mucous membranes of the eyes and nose during activities such as bathing [14, 41]. Globally, heavy rainfall and flooding are associated with leptospirosis outbreaks in overcrowded locations with deficient waste disposal and poor sanitation [41, 42]. These conditions prevail in Nigeria among socioeconomically disadvantaged communities living in shanty towns, squatter settlements and relief camps [43]. Zoonotic bacterial agents like *Salmonella*, *Campylobacter*, *Shigella*, *Yersinia* and *Listeria* may also be acquired from contact with animals, their dung and droppings, as well as via indirect transmission by ingesting contaminated food [3]. Although known to occur predominantly in temperate zones, sporadic infections with pathogenic serotypes of food-borne *Yersinia enterolitica* as well as the rare *Y. pseudotuberculosis* have been reported in Nigeria [20]. However, aspects of the epidemiology of food-borne yersiniosis in developing countries, such as contamination routes in food, remain poorly understood and require clarification [21].

While leptospirosis may also be acquired through food [14] *Salmonella* and *Campylobacter* are regarded as the leading and most frequent zoonotic agents of human food-borne bacterial gastroenteritis in both developing and developed regions globally. Research performed on food products from markets in the Nigerian States of Sokoto, Plateau and Oyo identified bacteria of both genera to be associated with, and commonly transmitted via, contamination of poultry meat and eggs [3, 22, 24, 44]. A recent investigation in the north-east of the country also identified vegetables as a potential source of salmonellosis transmission, corroborating reports of increasing frequency of *Salmonella* outbreaks elsewhere in the world [28].

Consumption of raw or unpasteurized milk constitutes an important transmission route for *Campylobacter spp.*, *C. burnetii* and *Brucella spp.* [3, 24, 29]. In Nigeria, *C. jejuni* was quite recently isolated from raw cow's milk in Sokoto [45], while shedding of *C. burnetii* was detected in milk from cattle in Zaria in the 1980s [46–48]. Q fever is a devastating zoonotic disease that is associated with dairy farming, especially of goats, even in industrialized nations like the Netherlands, where it was epidemic between 2007 and 2010 [3, 49]. Among Fulani pastoralists in Nigeria it is important to assess the risk of *C. burnetii* infection due to Q fever outbreaks [50–52].

Inhalation of aerosolized organisms, one of the ways to contract the plague-causing *Y. pestis* that is endemic to Africa, is also regarded as the most important transmission route for *C. burnetii* infection in humans [53, 54]. Aerosols containing *C. burnetii* result from infected animals shedding bacteria, usually during parturition and lactation, which are inhaled from placental fluid, vaginal mucus, milk, urine and environmental dust [48, 49]. Q fever contracted by humans inhaling contaminated aerosols or ingesting raw milk or raw milk products has been reported elsewhere but not yet in Nigeria [54, 55]. A nationwide assessment of the risk of *C. burnetii* contamination of aerosols and dairy products may be justified in light of the fact that 90% of milk produced in rural areas is consumed raw [13].

Q fever poses a chronic health risk to immunocompromised individuals [48]. Immunosuppression from such varied causes as cancer treatment, pregnancy, organ transplant, diabetes, alcoholism and even infancy is also an important risk factor for other bacterial zoonoses including salmonellosis, bovine tuberculosis and bartonellosis, with *Salmonella* being a leading cause of bacteremia in this at-risk population across sub-Saharan Africa [3, 10, 26, 33, 56].

2.2 Animal reservoirs and the potential role of arthropods as transmission vectors

Livestock and animal reservoirs are recognized to contribute substantially to the continued transmission of bacterial zoonoses. This involvement ranges from passive to active roles including passive transmission of infection through bites and scratches, contamination of the environment and active transmission as vectors [3, 41, 57, 58]. The widespread distribution of zoonotic pathogens in domestic and wild animal populations represents a large reservoir of these disease-causing agents. Consequently, there is a perpetually high risk of infection between infected and susceptible animals with the potential for spread to human hosts [13].

It is estimated that approximately 20% of animal bites or scratches become infected, which is an important transmission route to humans for *Bartonella henselae*, the causative agent of cat-scratch disease. This is also transmitted by cat fleas (*Ctenocephalides felis*) that are found on both cats and dogs [3, 53, 59]. Cats are under-studied as potential reservoirs of locally acquired *Bartonella* infection despite their relative popularity as companion animals and the frequent occurrence of strays [60, 61] even in hospital premises in northern Nigeria [62]. However, a first report of bats as reservoirs of *Bartonella* in Nigeria identified four species as well as blood-feeding bat flies as possible contributors to local transmission of bartonellosis [7], similar to findings from Kenya, Ghana and Algeria [63–65]. While bats are thought to host numerous pathogens, most research has focused on viral zoonotic agents. Accordingly, the main aim of the recent survey overseen by the Nigerian Ministry of Health was to catalog new and existing viruses in the bat population [7, 66]. These flying mammals live near humans in many communities in Nigeria, where they are used for food, cultural practices and rituals. They may therefore play hitherto unrecognized roles in transmission of *Bartonella* and other zoonotic bacterial agents [7].

The past decade has seen reports of fleas, which are commonly known to transmit *Y. pestis* plague and likely contribute to the transmission of zoonotic pathogens such as *Rickettsia typhi*, *R. felis* and *B. henselae* [53, 67]. Therefore, it is necessary to investigate this hematophagous insect vector in Nigeria, a location where information about the possible role of fleas in zoonotic transmission is scarce. Conducted in 2011, the first known examination of rodents and their ectoparasites for *Bartonella* in Nigeria detected species in fleas, ticks and earwigs; some isolates represent known strains while others are of uncertain identity and require further characterization and evaluation for possible pathogenicity [34]. Meanwhile, human fleas (*Pulex irritans*), which have been found to infest Nigerian pets [68], and cat fleas have each been linked with recently re-emerged *Bartonella quintana* infections in some developed countries [53]. Cat fleas and several other flea species are also considered to be major reservoirs and biological vectors of *R. felis*, capable of transmitting this pathogen horizontally and vertically. However, conflicting reports from Senegal suggest that, despite the high prevalence of human infection, cat fleas do not contribute to local transmission of *R. felis* [53, 69]. Canine fleas such as *Ctenocephalides canis*, associated with transmission of *B. henselae* in other global regions, have a high prevalence in Nigeria where pet dogs are ubiquitous and in close contact with humans, yet the potential role of this flea in transmitting zoonoses locally is not well understood [68, 70, 71]. It is also thought that any species of flea is capable of transmitting *Y. pestis* under suitable conditions, and that *P. irritans* may play a crucial role in the transmission of plague from person to person [53]. Often considered a mere nuisance because of prior reports of vector incompetence for *Y. pestis*, cat fleas are suspected of causing an outbreak of plague in Uganda [53]. However, although human and other flea species are found on Nigerian pets there is currently no documented association between cat fleas and local transmission of *Y. pestis* [38].

In addition to hosting *Y. pestis*, rodents are reservoirs of *R. typhi*, the causative agent of murine typhus, as well as other zoonotic bacteria like *Bartonella* [32, 53]. *Y. pestis* has been detected in over 200 species of wild rodent in natural plague foci in Africa and across the globe [32, 53]. Small mammals such as rodents are common natural *Bartonella* reservoirs and close associations with humans due to conditions like overcrowding in rural communities enhance infection transmission [31, 33]. Rodents, particularly rats, are also widely recognized as prominent reservoirs of *L. interrogans*, typically spreading leptospirosis via their infected urine [42]. A variety of wild and domestic animals that are considered reservoirs of *Leptospira* have been extensively studied for leptospirosis in Nigeria. Dogs, cattle, pigs, sheep and goats are recognized to excrete leptospirochetes in their urine, thereby contaminating the environment for many months or even years after infection [19, 39, 42]. Yet, in Nigeria very little effort has been made to investigate the contribution of rodents to the epidemiology of this disease, with the last known report being published in 1990 [42, 72].

Livestock are principal reservoirs of zoonotic infections such as brucellosis and Q fever, with ruminants being the main source for transmission to humans [29, 48, 55]. For food-borne zoonotic pathogens like *Y. pseudotuberculosis* and *Y. enterocolitica*, pigs, sheep, goats and cattle are the main reservoirs of the pathogenic serotypes causing human infection in Nigeria [20]. *C. jejuni* and other human campylobacteriosis agents are also food-borne bacteria for which chicken has frequently been identified in Nigeria and elsewhere as a common reservoir [23, 24]. A higher prevalence of *C. burnetii* was observed in feeding *Rhipicephalus evertsi* ticks than in questing ticks collected from cattle in Oyo State, indicating that cows may be reservoirs of Q fever in Nigeria [30]. Wild birds, dogs, cats and monkeys are also natural reservoirs of *Campylobacter*, with certain species showing association with specific animal hosts [23]. The increasing consumption of camel meat and its other products in northern Nigeria prompted investigation that identified camels as potential reservoirs of *Campylobacter* zoonosis [23]. Genomic analysis of *S. enterica* Eko isolates collected from various sources in Nigeria also demonstrated an association between camels and non-typhoidal *Salmonella* zoonoses, implicating camels, together with cattle, as a principal reservoir for infection of humans [27]. In low-income nations, where sources and routes of transmission of salmonellosis are poorly defined, common food-producing animals are considered to be major reservoirs of *Salmonella*. An example is that of poultry in Nigeria, the studies on which corroborated research performed elsewhere in identifying chickens as a major reservoir of a broad range of *Salmonella* serotypes such as Hadar known to colonize flocks [26, 28]. However, transmission of *Salmonella* has also been linked to pet and indoor-dwelling reptiles such as wall geckos in Nigeria and worldwide, pointing to a potential role for captive reptiles as reservoirs of disease [25]. A pet lizard was implicated as the source in the first report of human infection with *S. enterica* Apapa [73]. Infections of Apapa and other rare serotypes such as Jukestown, Mouschaui and Oritamerin were identified in Ibadan, where these bacteria were not detected in chickens screened for salmonellosis. This suggests local transmission via unverified sources of infection such as household lizards, as these serovars have previously been associated with reptiles and amphibians [25].

The number of known animal reservoirs and vectors of *Bartonella* also continues to increase; as with fleas, other hematophagous arthropods such as sand flies, lice, mites and ticks transmit bartonelloses between the reservoir and final mammalian host, including humans [3, 34]. Tick-borne bacteria and other pathogens are recognized as significant causative agents of human and animal disease [33]. Considered a carrier of infectious disease second only to mosquitoes [33, 74], ticks were identified as a potential vector of Q fever in the 1930s following the first isolation of *C. burnetii* from *Dermacentor andersoni*, the Rocky Mountain wood tick [55]. Because of the frequent detection of *C. burnetii* in ticks collected from the wild as well as experimental evidence of their vectorial capacity, ticks are now considered to act as vectors of

Q fever transmission [55]. The tropical bont tick, *Amblyomma variegatum*, is adept at supporting transmission of *C. burnetii*, for which it is considered a reservoir, as well as of *R. africae*, in Nigeria and Uganda [54, 75]. The largest tick species in Nigeria, *A. variegatum*, is the most common, providing a significant risk of Q fever transmission in Nassarawa, Oyo and Plateau States, where *C. burnetii* has been isolated from field-sampled ticks [54]. Detection of *C. burnetii* in ticks should be carefully interpreted until a method to directly distinguish between *C. burnetii* and *Coxiella*-like bacteria is developed. However, while following currently recommended procedures for screening for *C. burnetii*, these findings point to a role for tick reservoirs in transmitting Q fever in Nigeria [55].

Tick-borne rickettsiosis also occurs frequently in West Africa and *R. conorii israelensis*, the etiological agent of Mediterranean Spotted Fever which has been reported in Senegal [76], was first detected in Nigeria in the brown dog tick, *Rhipicephalus sanguineus* [34]. *R. africae*, the cause of African tick-bite fever, was identified in the cattle tick, *Rhipicephalus microplus*, from Nigeria in a study screening fed and questing ticks [30]. This rickettsial species is often associated with *Amblyomma* ticks and less commonly with other possible vectors including *Rhipicephalus annulatus* [77]. *R. africae* was isolated from feeding ticks only, so was likely acquired by ingesting blood from an infected host [30, 77–79]. From these reports it is unclear which tick species are potential vectors and thus further elucidation of their vector competence is required. A further Nigerian study in which dogs and brown dog ticks were free of *R. africae* may indicate a specific association between zoonotic bacteria and ticks of cattle and game animals [33], as reported in South Africa [80]. Detection of *Rickettsia massilae* in unfed ticks but not in their cattle hosts implies that ticks serve as both an important vector and reservoir of this pathogen in Nigeria [30]. Similarly, in Plateau State, *Bartonella spp.* was identified in *R. sanguineus* but not in rodent hosts, suggesting that the brown dog tick, whose role in transmission of *Bartonella* has not been previously shown, may be a local reservoir [33].

Other agents of bacterial zoonoses that have been associated with ticks in Nigeria include *Candidatus N. mikurensis* and *A. platys*, which were first detected in dogs, *Ehrlichia spp*., and a possibly novel form of the *Borrelia burgdorferi sensu lato* group that differs from known forms and which is associated with the *Rhipicephalus* ticks that can parasitize humans [30, 34, 68]. Comparing prevalence of pathogen bacteria in Nigerian ticks reiterates that detection in feeding ticks does not establish vectorial competence, i.e., the capacity of a tick to acquire, maintain, and transmit a bacterial species [30]. This highlights the need to demonstrate experimentally the vector capacity of ticks to sustain transstadial transmissibility of major zoonotic bacterial pathogens [30].

While the *in vitro* vector capacity of ticks, from which *Leptospira spp.* were isolated, was demonstrated several years ago, a link between arthropods and transmission of leptospirosis is not widely acknowledged [39, 81]. However, *Leptospira* was detected recently in *Ixodes* ticks from a wetland in Poland, eastern Europe [81]. This hints at a switch of *Leptospira*, aided by environmental fluxes, to adapt to novel hosts and maintain transmission through them, as previously documented for *L. interrogans* Hardjo serovar [41]. This finding requires confirmation from other global locations where ticks are recognized to contribute to transmission of bacterial zoonoses. However, *Ixodes* ticks of medical and veterinary importance are not a common presence in those regions of Nigeria that are prone to flooding [33].

Recent research suggests that mosquito species have emerged as transmission vectors for *R. felis* in West Africa. *R. felis* was detected in the tiger mosquito, *Aedes albopictus*, in Gabon, which lies to the south of Nigeria, at a similar infection load as found in the cat flea, *Ctenocephalides felis*, currently considered as the primary vector [82]. An invasive species to Nigeria, *Ae. albopictus* is now dominant over the native yellow fever mosquito, *Ae. aegypti*; first discovered in Delta State, analysis suggests a broader distribution across the southern part of the country [83]. Although originally identified in Nigeria in 1991 and first reported in Gabon as recently as 2006, the role of *Ae. albopictus* in arbovirus transmission is a major focus of investigation in Nigeria [83], yet its possible association with *R. felis* is less of a research priority. In Cote d'Ivoire, Gabon and Senegal, West African countries in which *Ae. albopictus* is not known to occur, the major malaria vector in Africa, *Anopheles gambiae*, presents a threat of rickettsial infection as *R. felis* and a new *Rickettsia* species were detected in *An. gambiae* and also *An. melas* [84].

Mosquito transmission may be implicated in the high risk of *R. felis* infection that has been reported in Senegal, where fleas are not involved [36, 69]. However, the possible role of mosquito species in transmitting rickettsial zoonoses in Nigeria remains poorly understood or not described. This also applies to other arthropods, particularly the housefly, *Musca domestica*, which has been identified as a potential mechanical vector able to transmit zoonotic infectious agents such as *C. burnetii* and *Campylobacter* in other parts of the world [58, 85].

2.3 Zoonosis surveillance and public health interventions

Infection rates in surveillance indicators such as arthropods and other host animals are commonly used to determine the risk of local transmission of pathogens to humans. Thus, within a defined area, the abundance and distribution of ticks and other hematophagous vectors are considered determinants of the epidemiology of vector-borne infections [33, 86]. Nigerian investigations showed that ongoing transmission of emerging and re-emerging bacterial zoonoses is associated with several animal reservoirs and vectors, while preliminary assessment of the risk of infection has also been made [13]. Human infection data are also a valuable surveillance indicator of infection risk [86]. However, in Nigeria this information is vanishingly scarce for bacterial zoonoses such as brucellosis, of which little is known about its prevalence. Further studies are needed to provide comprehensive profiling of clinical cases [13, 29]. Serological evidence of human brucellosis has been recorded but no details are available on the isolation of *Brucella* from patients in Nigeria [29].

Estimates of vector-borne infectious disease burden in low- and middle-income countries focus primarily on malaria and dengue, while zoonotic bacterial infections are largely ignored [8]. This is irrespective of reports from Nigeria justifying an assessment of the human disease burden imposed by *C. burnetii*, *R. conorii israelensis* and other zoonotic pathogens, plus a lack of attention to the public health impacts related to different vectors and animal reservoirs [30, 33]. This neglect of zoonotic bacterial infections is explained partly by under-reporting resulting in a reduced estimation of their disease burden and health impacts, which downgrades their relevance to politicians, policymakers and other interested parties [12]. In Nigeria, brucellosis is often confused with malaria [29], which frequently occurs in the reporting of bacterial zoonoses in other malaria-endemic areas [87]. Recent research conducted in malaria-endemic northern Tanzania showed that leptospirosis, brucellosis, rickettsioses and Q fever are often excluded or misdiagnosed as the parasitic disease [5]. After the gradual reduction of malaria incidence in sub-Saharan Africa this century, there is raised awareness of bacterial zoonoses as significant causes of FUO [5, 88, 89].

In the capital city of Nigeria, the centrally located Abuja, where historical overdiagnosis of malaria is suspected, non-typhoidal *Salmonella* infections were reported in the etiological diagnosis of febrile illnesses [90]. In contrast, for a case of FUO in southeast Nigeria, plausible causes were overlooked in favor of a presumptive malaria diagnosis, a practice common in this region that is also reported for management of febrile pediatric cases [91, 92]. Patients in Africa infected with bacterial zoonoses are likely to be discharged from hospital without receiving a correct diagnosis and thus the appropriate specific treatment. Focus on a wide range of potential causes of FUO, especially zoonotic infections, has been recommended for patient management and disease control in resource-limited settings [5].

While public health interventions for zoonotic infections in Nigeria have been proposed, prioritizing a disease for investment and funding will depend on impact assessments on both humans and animals [12, 13]. Initial reports identified how important joint efforts of medical and veterinary professionals are to controlling zoonoses that affect Nigerian public health and animal welfare [1]. Subsequently, the key role of the Ministries of Agriculture, Health and Information to promote the health of human and animal populations was emphasized [10, 13]. The complex interdependent relationships between human, animal and environmental health have given rise to the concept of 'One Health'. This promotes collaboration of experts from diverse fields, such as physicians, veterinarians and environmentalists, working at state, national and international levels to achieve improved public health outcomes [2]. Despite growing global support for countries to embrace a One Health approach, in Nigeria the interdisciplinary similarities, especially between clinical and veterinary medicine, have not yet been recognized. This remains a major challenge to progress in addressing zoonotic diseases in the country despite increasing awareness of misdiagnosed undifferentiated fever [2, 13]. In 2009, the US Centers for Disease Control and Prevention launched the Animal-Human Interface Project (AHIP), providing technical training to facilitate progress on One Health in Nigeria [66]. Several collaborative projects have been promoted by AHIP together with partner agencies in Nigeria to investigate a wide range of zoonoses; however, attention has mainly focused on viral diseases. This may reflect the assertion that zoonotic viruses have the potential to influence stronger political and economic responses, as exemplified by recent Ebola outbreaks in Nigeria and the Democratic Republic of the Congo [93, 94].

A key recommendation of the One Health strategy for food-borne zoonoses is on-farm intervention. This includes routine vaccinations, immunostimulants and probiotic feed additives to manage animal health, as well as implementing animal welfare policies and measures to limit antibiotic resistance [3]. However, the successful adoption of these interventions in Nigeria is restricted by sustainability issues resulting from the discontinuation of disease control programs [13]. Furthermore, culling livestock and compensating farmers, a strategy that has helped to control zoonoses in industrialized nations, has not proved effective in Nigeria. This is because farmers, especially Fulani pastoralists, are unwilling to cooperate when infectious disease control involves the intentional loss of their herds [13]. However, changing lifestyles among settled Fulani communities, including healthcare attitudes and practices, may lead to greater receptivity of this influential group to interventions in future [51].

Among food-borne zoonoses such as salmonellosis conspicuous antimicrobial resistance of public health concern has been reported in Nigeria [25, 95]. Curbing the indiscriminate use of antibiotics as animal growth promoters that is commonly practiced requires the imposition of strict regulations. *S. enterica* Typhimurium isolates bearing close similarity to the multidrug-resistant ST313 strain that circulates in sub-Saharan Africa, as well as other strains resistant to tetracycline and sulfamethoxazole, have been identified in Ibadan [25]. This is attributed to the non-selective use of antibiotics at therapeutic and sub-therapeutic doses, which was observed in cattle examined in the same location where residual doses of oxytetracycline and penicillin-G were found [96]. Of associated concern, an alarming trend in the use of fluoroquinolones, tetracyclines, beta-lactams/aminoglycosides and macrolides for questionable purposes including disease management and growth promotion of livestock was recently highlighted for southwest Nigeria [95]. Meanwhile, other countries led by the United States have banned quinolones as a growth promoter in poultry feed due to the public health impact of pharmaceuticals used to treat both human and infections [3, 95]. In Nigeria, there are no strict laws governing antibiotic residues in animal tissues, while local food and drug regulatory authorities do not pay much attention to veterinary drug safety regulations [97].

Vector-borne diseases are also an important target of the One Health approach. It is expected that better national surveillance and reporting will improve disease control strategies, whereby clinicians play an important role in the effective management of vector-borne zoonoses with enhanced differential diagnoses [3]. The multiple causes of fever are difficult to distinguish clinically and hence many cases of FUO in low-resource contexts may be attributed to either lack of access to or limited provision of suitable medical microbiology laboratory services [8]. As an example, it was reported that Nigerian abattoir workers who eventually received a correct diagnosis of *Brucella* infection frequently complained of continued treatment for malaria despite their condition failing to improve [29]. It is evident that clinicians often lack information on the local epidemiology of causes of severe febrile illness. Consequently, internationally set management guidelines and disease control programs currently have insufficient data to set local priorities for prevention [8].

In sub-Sahara Africa, where hospitals and clinics typically are not readily accessible to affected people, accurate statistics on morbidity and mortality resulting from bacterial zoonoses are difficult to obtain [12]. Food-borne yersiniosis caused by the pathogenic *Y. enterolitica* that is commonly found in developed nations has been associated with chronic gastrointestinal illness, glomerulopathy and other disease symptoms in Nigerians [21, 98]. While *Bartonella spp.* are linked with endocarditis and neuroretinitis in Peru [32], for identical strains isolated in Nigeria a similar association to human disease has yet to be made [34]. In Senegal, where there are lower rates of detection of *C. burnetii* in reservoir cattle than those in Nigeria, seroprevalence rates in humans are as high as 51% [48], suggesting that these may be even surpassed in Nigeria [30]; however, this requires to be substantiated through further investigation. While a case of human leptospirosis recently occurred in Plateau State, no survey of leptospirosis as the cause of febrile illness has been conducted in Nigeria [42]. In 2006, the zoonotic bacterial infections leptospirosis, brucellosis, bovine tuberculosis, campylobacteriosis and salmonellosis were acknowledged as less recognized and under-reported [99]. The true extent to which these zoonoses exert an impact on health, especially at the population level, is unknown. In the following decade, the situation remained generally unchanged for most of these diseases, including brucellosis [29]. Therefore, the underestimation of zoonotic bacterial pathogens in Nigeria contributes to a dearth of integrated approaches to preventing morbidity and mortality from febrile illnesses. For example, this relative neglect stands in stark contrast to pneumonia and diarrhea, each of which is the focus of coordinated global control and prevention initiatives across most of its pathogen range [4, 5].

Determining the spatiotemporal distribution of an infectious disease is an important step in planning and implementing effective infection control and prevention measures [100]. However, in developing countries coordinated epidemiological systems for national surveillance of zoonotic infections are generally inadequate despite indications of a substantial burden of disease [22, 26]. The first comprehensive laboratory-based surveillance of human and animal salmonellosis in Nigeria was targeted at the north-east of the country [101], while another more recent attempt that employed whole genome sequencing to identify sources of *Salmonella* infection from isolates collected across Nigeria was focused solely on the *S. enterica* Eko serovar [27]. Reports from the country on human brucellosis similarly focus on standard at-risk populations and thus ignore other potentially susceptible groups. As a result, a century since its initial identification in Nigeria, little is still known about *Brucella* in regard to accurately assessing its zoonotic potential and hence informing establishment of appropriate control measures [29].

Many endemic diseases have increased in global incidence in the past two decades and a large number of vector-borne infections have also emerged in new regions [3]. For Nigeria, this growing public health concern underscores the need for up-to-date, accurate information on bacterial zoonoses, particularly with respect to arthropod-borne zoonotic pathogens that have recently emerged in novel vectors, such as *R. felis* in mosquitoes [68]. There is a correlation between the epidemiology of *R. felis* infection and increased risk of dengue in sub-Saharan Africa but not in other regions [78]. Mosquito species identified as potential vectors of *R. felis* in other West African countries, and which may be responsible for its transmission in Senegal [84], are known to be endemic to Nigeria [69, 82–84]. Although human rickettsial infections have yet to be confirmed in Nigeria, as a precautionary measure they are highlighted as a source of potential disease for travelers to the country [102]. Other pathogenic agents of bacterial zoonoses such as *Candidatus N. mikurensis* and *Y. pseudotuberculosis* were described recently for the first time in Nigeria [20, 33], which indicates an extension of their respective geographic ranges into the country.

The risk of contracting zoonotic bacterial infections is elevated among rural communities and for individuals who otherwise come into close contact with livestock or wild animals. Unfortunately, zoonoses that mainly affect subsistence farmers and low-income residents of regional and remote regions do not have a designated control or prevention scheme within Nigeria's national healthcare program [12, 13]. Misreporting of cases and undervaluation of the clinical impact of a disease are factors for a lack of prioritized investment in tailored health interventions [12]. Applying a global burden of human disease methodology, Nigerian policymakers rely on unsubstantiated, incomplete data from other regions, an extrapolation that contributes to the systematic depreciation of zoonotic diseases nationwide [12]. The consequent paucity of resource commitment to public health issues by Nigeria and other developing countries poses a continuing challenge for One Health interdisciplinary collaborations and partnerships to enhance public health surveillance and disease control [13].

As an alternative criterion to total disease burden, appraising the cost-effectiveness of an intervention is a way to identify investment priorities for infection control [103]. The existence of multiple reservoir hosts is highlighted as a major hindrance to the elimination of zoonoses in Nigeria. Thus, interventions primarily targeting animal reservoirs and accompanied by promoting national public awareness are considered cost-effective strategies to constrain zoonotic bacterial and non-bacterial diseases [10, 13]. Investing funds in monitoring and treating animal populations is rarely supported strongly in most developing countries despite the potential benefits of improving food security and reducing poverty [12]. Interventions for zoonotic diseases may seem expensive in proportion to the public health benefits *per se*. Evidence of the burden to communities and the cost-effectiveness of integrated control would strengthen the case for a One Health approach to endemic zoonotic diseases [12]. It is argued that by investing in animal health interventions and veterinary care the exposure of a population to locally endemic zoonotic diseases is commensurately reduced [13, 104].

The rewards of a multidisciplinary analysis that covers health and economic factors will easily exceed the outlay and enable the health sector to present a case to policymakers based not on the impact on disability-adjusted life years but rather on the rate of return on public and private investment [12]. Hence, it is advocated that in Nigeria interventions against zoonotic infections should be viewed as a human capital asset and as integral to a poverty reduction plan [12].

3. Future directions

In order to enhance the security of human and animal health in Nigeria, cost-effective strategies are needed to raise the prioritization of bacterial zoonoses in health policies and to encourage investment in health interventions [9]. Current epidemiological surveillance of zoonotic bacterial infections across the country is incomplete, a situation that hinders development of a One Health program. This is an impediment to interdisciplinary collaboration between qualified professionals including environmentalists, veterinarians and clinicians. While different species and strains of common and rare pathogenic bacteria have been identified in vectors and reservoir animals in Nigeria, little is known about their potential impact on human health. Indeed, data on human infection do not exist for some zoonotic diseases. Recent research revealing the emergence of several zoonotic bacterial pathogens in previously unknown vectors and in new geographic locations demands a re-evaluation of their formally recognized national distributions. The knowledge gap regarding bacterial zoonoses in Nigeria is significant, closing of which is critical to the future success of control and preventive interventions. Implementing these public health measures will likely reduce local incidence of FUO.

Author contributions

Both authors contributed significantly to preparing and writing this chapter.

Funding statement

No specific funding was received for this work.

Competing interests

No conflicts of interest declared.

Author details

Andrew W. Taylor-Robinson[1,2,3,4*] and Olaitan O. Omitola[5]

1 College of Health Sciences, VinUniversity, Hanoi, Vietnam

2 Center for Global Health, University of Pennsylvania, Philadelphia, USA

3 School of Health, Medical and Applied Sciences, Central Queensland University, Brisbane, Australia

4 College of Health and Human Sciences, Charles Darwin University, Casuarina, Australia

5 Department of Pure and Applied Zoology, Federal University of Agriculture, Abeokuta, Nigeria

*Address all correspondence to: andrew.tr@vinuni.edu.vn

References

[1] Coker AO, Isokpehi RD, Thomas BN, Fagbenro-Beyioku AF, Omilabu SA. Zoonotic infections in Nigeria: Overview from a medical perspective. Acta Tropica. 2000;**76**(1):59-63

[2] Yakubu Y, Junaidu AU, Magaji AA, Salihu MD, Mahmuda A, Shehu S. One health—The fate of public health in Nigeria. Asian Journal of Medical Sciences. 2011;**3**(1):47-49

[3] Cantas L, Suer K. Review: The important bacterial zoonoses in "*One Health*" concept. Frontiers in Public Health. 2014;**2**:144

[4] Ngutor KS. A multidisciplinary approach in the control of zoonoses in Nigeria. Journal of Veterinary Advances. 2012;**2**(12):557-567

[5] Crump JA, Morrissey AB, Nicholson WL, Massung RF, Stoddard RA, Galloway RL, et al. Etiology of severe non-malaria febrile illness in northern Tanzania: A prospective cohort study. PLoS Neglected Tropical Diseases. 2013;**7**(7):e2324

[6] Oladosu OO, Oyibo WA. Overdiagnosis and overtreatment of malaria in children that presented with fever in Lagos, Nigeria. ISRN Infectious Diseases. 2013;**2013**:914675

[7] Kamani J, Baneth G, Mitchell M, Mumcuoglu KY, Gutiérrez R, Harrus S. *Bartonella* species in bats (Chiroptera) and bat flies (Nycteribiidae) from Nigeria, West Africa. Vector Borne Zoonotic Diseases. 2014;**14**(9): 625-632

[8] Prasad N, Murdoch DR, Reyburn H, Crump JA. Etiology of severe febrile illness in low- and middle-income countries: A systematic review. PLoS One. 2015;**10**(6):e0127962

[9] Omitola OO, Taylor-Robinson AW. Emerging and re-emerging bacterial zoonoses in Nigeria: Current preventive measures and future approaches to intervention. Heliyon. 2020;**6**:e04095

[10] Musa OI, Akanbi AA II, Bolarinwa OA. Epidemiology and control of zoonotic infections in Nigeria. African Scientist. 2007;**8**(2):109-114

[11] Isere EE, Fatiregun AA, Ajay IO. An overview of disease surveillance and notification system in Nigeria and the roles of clinicians in disease outbreak prevention and control. Nigerian Medical Journal. 2015;**56**(3):161-168

[12] Welburn SC, Beange I, Ducrotoy MJ, Okello AL. The neglected zoonoses—The case for integrated control and advocacy. Clinical Microbiology and Infection. 2015;**21**(5):433-443

[13] Ehizibolo DO, Ehizibolo PO, Ehizibolo EE, Sugun MY, Idachaba SE. The control of neglected zoonotic diseases in Nigeria through animal intervention. African Journal of Biomedical Research. 2011;**14**(1):81-88

[14] Abiayi EA, Inabo HI, Jatau ED, Makinde AA, Sar TT, Ugbe DA, et al. Knowledge, attitudes, risk factors and practices (KARP) that favor *Leptospira* infection among abattoir workers in north Central Nigeria. Asian Journal of Epidemiology. 2015;**8**(4):104-113

[15] Awosanya EJ, Nguku P, Oyemakinde A, Omobowale O. Factors associated with probable cluster of leptospirosis among kennel workers in

Abuja, Nigeria. Pan African Medical Journal. 2013;**16**(1):144

[16] Ezeh AO, Adesiyun AA, Addo PB, Ellis WA, Makinde AA, Bello CS. Serological and cultural examination for human leptospirosis in Plateau state, Nigeria. Central African Journal of Medicine. 1991;**37**(1):11-15

[17] Onyemelukwe NF. A serological survey for leptospirosis in the Enugu area of eastern Nigeria among people at occupational risk. The Journal of Tropical Medicine and Hygiene. 1993;**96**(5):301-304

[18] Agunloye CA, Alabi FO, Odemuyiwa SO, Olaleye OD. Leptospirosis in Nigerians: A seroepidemiological survey. The Indian Veterinary Journal. 2001;**78**(5):371-375

[19] Brown K, Prescott J. Leptospirosis in the family dog: A public health perspective. Canadian Medical Association Journal. 2008;**178**(4):399-401

[20] Okwori AEJ, Martínez PO, Fredriksson-Ahomaa M, Agina SE, Korkeala H. Pathogenic *Yersinia enterocolitica* 2/O:9 and *Yersinia pseudotuberculosis* 1/O:1 strains isolated from human and non-human sources in the Plateau state of Nigeria. Food Microbiology. 2009;**26**(8):872-875

[21] Rahman A, Bonny TS, Stonsaovapak S, Ananchaipattana C. *Yersinia enterocolitica*: Epidemiological studies and outbreaks. J. Pathog. 2011;**2011**:239391

[22] Coker AO, Isokpehi RD, Thomas BN, Amisu KO, Obi CL. Human campylobacteriosis in developing countries. Emerging Infectious Diseases. 2002;**8**(3):237-244

[23] Salihu MD, Junaidu AU, Abubakar MB, Magaji AA, Mohammed LG. Isolation and characterization of *Campylobacter* species from camel (*Camelus dromedarius*) in Sokoto state, northwestern Nigeria. International Journal of Animal and Veterinary Advances. 2009;**1**(1):25-27

[24] Olatoye O, Ogunsemoyin O. Prevalence and antibiotics resistance of *Campylobacter jejuni* in retail chickens in Oyo state, Nigeria. Food Science and Quality Management. 2016;**48**(1):7-11

[25] Fashae K, Ogunsola F, Aarestrup FM, Hendriksen RS. Antimicrobial susceptibility and serovars of *salmonella* from chickens and humans in Ibadan, Nigeria. Journal of Infection in Developing Countries. 2010;**4**(8):484-494

[26] Kagambèga A, Lienemann T, Aulu L, Traoré AS, Barro N. Prevalence and characterization of *Salmonella enterica* from the feces of cattle, poultry, swine and hedgehogs in Burkina Faso and their comparison to human *Salmonella* isolates. BMC Microbiology. 2013;**13**:253

[27] Leekitcharoenphon P, Raufu I, Nielsen MT, Rosenqvist Lund BS, Ameh JA, Ambali AG, et al. Investigating *Salmonella* Eko from various sources in Nigeria by whole genome sequencing to identify the source of human infections. PLoS One. 2016;**11**(5):e0156212

[28] Raufu IA, Zongur L, Lawan FA, Bello HS, Adamu MS, et al. Prevalence and antimicrobial profiles of *Salmonella* serovars from vegetables in Maiduguri, north eastern Nigeria. Sokoto Journal of Veterinary Sciences. 2014;**12**(1):23-28

[29] Ducrotoy MJ, Bertu WJ, Ocholi RA, Gusi AM, Bryssinckx W, Welburn S, et al. Brucellosis as an emerging threat in developing economies: Lessons from Nigeria. PLoS Neglected Tropical Diseases. 2014;**8**(7):e3008

[30] Reye AL, Arinola OG, Hübschen JM, Muller CP. Pathogen prevalence in ticks collected from the vegetation and livestock in Nigeria. Applied and Environmental Microbiology. 2012;**78**(8):2562-2568

[31] Martin-Alonso A, Soto M, Foronda P, Aguilar E, Bonnet G, Pacheco R, et al. *Bartonella* spp. and *Yersinia pestis* reservoirs, Cusco, Peru. Emerging Infectious Diseases. 2014;**20**(6):1069-1070

[32] Gutiérrez R, Krasnov B, Morick D, Gottlieb Y, Khokhlova IS, Harrus S. *Bartonella* infection in rodents and their flea ectoparasites: An overview. Vector Borne and Zoonotic Diseases. 2015;**15**(1):27-39

[33] Kamani J, Morick D, Mumcuoglu KY, Harrus S. Prevalence and diversity of *Bartonella* species in commensal rodents and ectoparasites from Nigeria, West Africa. PLOS Neglected Tropical Diseases. 2013;7(5):e2246

[34] Kamani J, Baneth G, Mumcuoglu KY, Waziri NE, Eyal O, Guthmann Y, et al. Molecular detection and characterization of tick-borne pathogens in dogs and ticks from Nigeria. PLoS Neglected Tropical Diseases. 2013;7(3):e2108

[35] Lorusso V, Wijnveld M, Majekodunmi AO, Dongkum C, Fajinmi A, Dogo AG, et al. Tick-borne pathogens of zoonotic and veterinary importance in Nigerian cattle. Parasites & Vectors. 2016;**9**:217

[36] Mediannikov O, Socolovschi C, Edouard S, Fenollar F, Mouffok N, Bassene H, et al. Common epidemiology of *Rickettsia felis* infection and malaria, Africa. Emerging Infectious Diseases. 2013;**19**(11):1775-1783

[37] de Silva AM, Fikrig E. Arthropod- and host-specific gene expression by *Borrelia burgdorferi*. The Journal of Clinical Investigation. 1997;**99**(3):377-379

[38] Neerinckx SB, Peterson AT, Gulinck H, Deckers J, Leirs H. Geographic distribution and ecological niche of plague in sub-Saharan Africa. International Journal of Health Geographics. 2008;7:54

[39] Luiz-Adrian JA. Leptospirosis: Identification and treatment in companion animals. Pacific Agriculture and Natural Resources. 2008;**15**(1):1-4

[40] Mwachui MA, Crump L, Hartskeerl R, Zinsstag J, Hattendorf J. Environmental and behavioural determinants of leptospirosis transmission: A systematic review. PLoS Neglected Tropical Diseases. 2015;**9**(9):e0003843

[41] Terpstra WJ. Historical perspectives in leptospirosis. Indian Journal of Medical Microbiology. 2006;**24**(4):316-320

[42] de Vries SG, Visser BJ, Nagel IM, Goris MGA, Hartskeerl RA, Grobusch MP. Leptospirosis in sub-Saharan Africa: A systematic review. International Journal of Infectious Diseases. 2014;**28**(1):47-64

[43] Ito EE, Egwunyenga AO. Schistosomiasis: The aftermath of 2012 floods in Delta state, southern Nigeria. Internal Medicine Journal. 2015;**22**(4):218-223

[44] Mai HM, Zahraddeen D, Qadeers MA, Bawa IA, Echeonwu IE. Investigation of some species of *Salmonella* in table eggs sold at different markets in Jos south, Plateau state, Nigeria. Global Advanced Research Journal of Microbiology. 2013;**2**(11):234-238

[45] Salihu MD, Junaidu AU, Magaji AA, Rabiu ZM. Study of *Campylobacter* in raw cow milk in Sokoto state, Nigeria. British Journal of Dairy Sciences. 2010;**1**(1):1-5

[46] Adesiyun AA, Jagun AG, Tekdek LB. *Coxiella burnetii* antibodies in some Nigerian dairy cows and their suckling calves. International Journal of Zoonoses. 1984;**11**(2):155-160

[47] Adesiyun AA, Jagun AG, Kwaga JK, Tekdek LB. Shedding of *Coxiella burnetii* in milk by Nigerian dairy and dual purposes cows. International Journal of Zoonoses. 1985;**12**(1):1-5

[48] Vanderburg S, Rubach MP, Halliday JEB, Cleaveland S, Reddy EA, Crump JA. Epidemiology of *Coxiella burnetii* infection in Africa: A OneHealth systematic review. PLoS Neglected Tropical Diseases. 2014;**8**(4):e2787

[49] Abbasi S, Farzan R, Momtaz H. Molecular detection of *Coxiella burnetii* in goat bulk milk samples in some provinces of Iran. African Journal of Biotechnology. 2011;**10**(80):18513-18515

[50] Köster HW, de Wolff J, Ikpo KP. Dairy Development Programme in Nigeria Baseline Report. Accelerating Agribusiness in Africa (AAA) Baseline Project. USA: International Fertilizer Development Center, Muscle Shoals; 2012

[51] Omotayo AM, Dipeolu MA, Ekpo UF. Health Consequences of Lifestyle Changes among Settled Fulani Pastoralists in South Western Nigeria. Ibadan, Nigeria: John Archers; 2005

[52] Saleh MK, Atala TK, Omokore DF, Ahmed B, Ali FS, Kajang GY. Performance of improved dairy cattle technologies among farmers in Northern Nigeria. Journal of Agricultural Extension. 2016;**20**(1):1-12

[53] Bitam I, Dittmar K, Parola P, Whiting MF, Raoult D. Fleas and flea-borne diseases. International Journal of Infectious Diseases. 2010;**14**(8):e667-e676

[54] Ogo NI, Fernández de Mera IG, Galindo RC, Okubanjo OO, Inuwa HM, Agbede RIS, et al. Genetic characterization of *Coxiella burnetii* in *Amblyomma variegatum* ticks from North-central Nigeria: Public health importance. Veterinary World. 2013;**6**(10):818-822

[55] Elsa J, Duron O, Séverine B, González-Acuña D, Sidi-Boumedine K. Molecular methods routinely used to detect *Coxiella burnetii* in ticks cross-react with *Coxiella*-like bacteria. Infection Ecology & Epidemiology. 2015;**5**:29230

[56] Berrian AM, Martínez-López B, Quan V, Conrad PA, van Rooyen J, Simpson GJG, et al. Risk factors for bacterial zoonotic pathogens in acutely febrile patients in Mpumalanga Province, South Africa. Zoonoses Public Health. 2019;**66**(5):458-469

[57] Rolain JM, Gouriet F, Brouqui P, Larrey D, Janbon F, Vene S, et al. Concomitant or consecutive infection with *Coxiella burnetii* and tickborne diseases. Clinical Infectious Diseases. 2005;**40**(1):82-88

[58] Nelder MP, Lloyd JE, Loftis AD, Reeves WK. *Coxiella burnetii* in wild-caught filth flies. Emerging Infectious Diseases. 2008;**14**(6):1002-1004

[59] Centers for Disease Control and Prevention. Cat-Scratch Disease (*Bartonella henselae* Infection). Healthy People: Healthy Pets; 2014. https://www.cdc.gov/healthypets/diseases/cat-scratch.html

[60] Sowemimo OA. Prevalence and intensity of gastrointestinal parasites of domestic cats in Ode—Irele and Oyo communities, Southwest Nigeria. Journal of Parasitology and Vector Biology. 2012;**4**(1):7-13

[61] Maryam BKY, Gana BA, Ahmed GY, Abubakar WM, Istifanus S. A survey of blood types of the domestic cat (*Felis catus*) in Maiduguri, North-eastern Nigeria. Journal of Veterinary Science & Technology. 2014;**5**(1):152

[62] Raji AA, Magaji AA, Bello MB, Lawal MD, Mamuda A, Yahaya MS. Prevalence of gastrointestinal parasites of stray cats: A case study of two hospitals in Sokoto Metropolis, Sokoto, Nigeria. Journal of Bacteriology and Parasitology. 2013;**4**(4):175

[63] Kosoy M, Bai Y, Lynch T, Kuzmin IV, Niezgoda M, Franka R, et al. *Bartonella* spp. in bats, Kenya. Emerging Infectious Diseases. 2010;**16**(1):1875-1881

[64] Billeter SA, Hayman DTS, Peel AJ, Baker K, Wood JL, Cunningham A, et al. *Bartonella* species in bat flies (Diptera: Nycteribiidae) from western Africa. Parasitology. 2012;**139**(3):324-329

[65] Leulmi H, Aouadi A, Bitam I, Bessas A, Benakhla A, Raoult D, et al. Detection of *Bartonella tamiae*, *Coxiella burnetii* and rickettsiae in arthropods and tissues from wild and domestic animals in northeastern Algeria. Parasites & Vectors. 2016;**9**:27

[66] Centers for Disease Control and Prevention. One Health and Zoonoses Activities at 17 Select International Locations. National Center for Emerging and Zoonotic Infectious Diseases. One Health Office; 2014. https://www.cdc.gov/ncezid/dhcpp/pdfs/annual-report.pdf

[67] Dobler G, Pfeffer M. Fleas as parasites of the family Canidae. Parasites & Vectors. 2011;**4**:139

[68] Ugbomoiko US, Ariza L, Heukelbach J. Parasites of importance for human health in Nigerian dogs: High prevalence and limited knowledge of pet owners. BMC Veterinary Research. 2008;**4**:49

[69] Diemea C, Bechaha Y, Socolovschia C, Audolya G, Berengera J, Faye O, et al. Transmission potential of *Rickettsia felis* infection by *Anopheles gambiae* mosquitoes. Proceedings of the National Academy of Sciences of the United States of America. 2015;**112**(26):8088-8093

[70] Chukwu CC. Prevalence of fleas on dogs in Anambra state of Nigeria. International Journal of Zoonoses. 1985;**12**(3):192-195

[71] Ishida C, Tsuneoka H, Iino H, Murakami K, Inokuma H, Ohnishi T, et al. *Bartonella henselae* infection in domestic cat and dog fleas. Kansenshōgaku Zasshi. 2001;**75**(2):133-136

[72] Ezeh AO, Addo PB, Adesiyun AA, Makinde AA, Bello CSS. Serological and bacteriological examination of rodents for leptospirosis in Plateau state, Nigeria. Bulletin of Animal Health and Production in Africa. 1990;**38**:359-360

[73] Cooke FJ, De Pinna E, Maguire C, Guha S, Pickard DJ, Farrington M, et al. First report of human infection with *Salmonella enterica* serovar Apapa resulting from exposure to a pet lizard. Journal of Clinical Microbiology. 2009;**47**(8):2672-2674

[74] Parola P, Raoult D. Ticks and tickborne bacterial diseases in humans: An emerging infectious threat. Clinical Infectious Diseases. 2001;**32**(6):897-928

[75] Lorusso V, Gruszka KA, Majekodunmi A, Igweh A, Welburn SC, Picozzi K. *Rickettsia africae* in

Amblyomma variegatum ticks, Uganda and Nigeria. Emerging Infectious Diseases. 2013;**19**(10):1705-1707

[76] Ratmanov P, Mediannikov O, Raoult D. Vectorborne diseases in West Africa: Geographic distribution and geospatial characteristics. Transactions of the Royal Society of Tropical Medicine and Hygiene. 2013;**107**(5):273-284

[77] Yssouf A, Socolovschi C, Kernif T, Temmam S, Lagadec E, Tortosa P, et al. First molecular detection of *Rickettsia africae* in ticks from the Union of the Comoros. Parasites & Vectors. 2014;**7**:444

[78] Mediannikov O, Diatta G, Zolia Y, Balde MC, Kohar H, Trape JF, et al. Tick-borne rickettsiae in Guinea and Liberia. Ticks and Tick-borne Diseases. 2012;**3**(1):43-48

[79] Portillo A, Pérez-Martínez L, Santibáñez S, Blanco JR, Ibarra V, Oteo JA. Detection of *Rickettsia africae* in *Rhipicephalus* (*Boophilus*) *decoloratus* ticks from the Republic of Botswana, South Africa. The American Journal of Tropical Medicine and Hygiene. 2007;**77**(2):376-377

[80] Frean J, Blumberg L, Ogunbanjo GA. Tick bite fever in South Africa. South African Family Practice. 2008;**50**(2):33-35

[81] Wójcik-Fatla A, Zajac V, Cisak E, Sroka J, Sawczyn A, Dutkiewicz J. Leptospirosis as a tick-borne disease? Detection of *Leptospira spp*. in *Ixodes ricinus* ticks in eastern Poland. Annals of Agricultural and Environmental Medicine. 2012;**19**(4):656-659

[82] Socolovschi C, Pagés F, Raoult D. *Rickettsia felis* in *Aedes albopictus* mosquitoes, Libreville, Gabon. Emerging Infectious Diseases. 2012;**18**(10):1687-1689

[83] Adeleke MA, Sam-Wobo SO, Garza-Hernandez JA, Oluwole AS, Mafiana CF, Reyes-Villanueva F, et al. Twenty-three years after the first record of *Aedes albopictus* in Nigeria: Its current distribution and potential epidemiological implications. African Entomology: Journal of the Entomological Society of Southern Africa. 2015;**23**(2):348-355

[84] Socolovschi C, Pagés F, Ndiath MO, Ratmanov P, Raoult D. *Rickettsia* species in African *anopheles* mosquitoes. PLoS One. 2012;**7**(10):e48254

[85] Nichols GL. Fly transmission of *Campylobacter*. Emerging Infectious Diseases. 2005;**11**(3):361-364

[86] Bustamante DM, Lord CC. Sources of error in the estimation of mosquito infection rates used to assess risk of arbovirus transmission. The American Journal of Tropical Medicine and Hygiene. 2010;**82**(6):1172-1184

[87] Omitola OO, Mogaji HO, Taylor-Robinson AW. Managing febrile illness in malaria-endemic areas: Developing novel diagnostics using host immunological signatures as surrogate markers of infection. Current Immunology Reviews. 2019;**15**(2): 202-206

[88] Bertherat E, Renaut A, Nabias R, Dubreuil G, Georges-Courbot MC. Leptospirosis and Ebola virus infection in five gold-panning villages in northeastern Gabon. The American Journal of Tropical Medicine and Hygiene. 1999;**60**(4):610-615

[89] Steinmann P, Bonfoh B, Péter O, Schelling E, Traoré M, Zinsstag J. Seroprevalence of Q fever in febrile individuals in Mali. Tropical Medicine & International Health. 2005;**10**(6):612-617

[90] Obaro S, Lawson L, Essen U, Ibrahim K, Brooks K, Otuneye A, et al. Community acquired bacteremia in young children from Central Nigeria—A pilot study. BMC Infectious Diseases. 2011;**11**:137

[91] Onodugo O, Iroezindu M. Fever of unknown origin in a Nigerian doctor: An unusual case. Internet Journal of Tropical Medicine. 2013;**9**(1):1-4

[92] Okoro CI, Chukwuocha UM, Nwakwuo GC, Ukaga CN. Presumptive diagnosis and treatment of malaria in febrile children in parts of South Eastern Nigeria. Journal of Infectious Diseases & Therapy. 2015;**3**(5):240

[93] Obilade TT. The political economy of the Ebola virus disease (EVD); taking individual and community ownership in the prevention and control of EVD. Healthcare. 2015;**3**(1):36-49

[94] Omoleke SA, Mohammed I, Saidu Y. Ebola viral disease in West Africa: A threat to global health, economy and political stability. Journal of Public Health in Africa. 2016;**7**(1):534

[95] Adesokan HK, Akanbi IO, Akanbi IM, Obaweda RA. Pattern of antimicrobial usage in livestock animals in South-Western Nigeria: The need for alternative plans. The Onderstepoort Journal of Veterinary Research. 2015;**82**(1):816

[96] Adesokan HK, Agada CA, Adetunji VO, Akanbi IM. Oxytetracycline and penicillin-G residues in cattle slaughtered in South-Western Nigeria: Implications for livestock disease management and public health. Journal of the South African Veterinary Association. 2013;**84**(1):E1-E5

[97] Omeiza GK, Ajayi IE, Ode OJ. Assessment of antimicrobial drug residues in beef in Abuja, the Federal Capital Territory, Nigeria. Veterinaria Italiana. 2012;**48**(3):283-289

[98] Awunor-Renner C, Lawande RV. *Yersinia* and chronic glomerulopathy in the savannah region of Nigeria. The British Medical Journal. 1982;**285**(6353):1464

[99] Adesiji YO, Fagbami AH. Epidemiology of bacterial zoonoses in Nigeria. Nigerian Journal of Health and Biomedical Sciences. 2006;**5**(1):98-104

[100] Smith DL, Dushoff J, McKenzie FE. The risk of a mosquito-borne infection in a heterogeneous environment. PLoS Biology. 2004;**2**(11):e368

[101] Raufu I, Bortolaia V, Svendsen CA, Ameh JA, Ambali AG, Aarestrup FM, et al. The first attempt of an active integrated laboratory-based *Salmonella* surveillance programme in the north-eastern region of Nigeria. Journal of Applied Microbiology. 2013;**115**(4):1059-1067

[102] Centers for Disease Control and Prevention. Travelers' Health: Health Information for Travelers to Nigeria. Division of Global Migration and Quarantine: Clinician View; 2016. http://wwwnc.cdc.gov/travel/destinations/clinician/none/nigeria

[103] Canning D. Priority setting and the 'neglected' tropical diseases. Transactions of the Royal Society of Tropical Medicine and Hygiene. 2006;**100**(6):499-504

[104] Elelu N, Aiyedun JO, Mohammed IG, Oludairo OO, Odetokun IA, Mohammed KM, et al. Neglected zoonotic diseases in Nigeria: Role of the public health veterinarian. The Pan African Medical Journal. 2019;**32**(1):36

Chapter 9

Neotropical Echinococcosis: A Review

Roy D. Meléndez

Abstract

Echinococcus vogeli (Rausch and Berstein, 1972) and *Echinococcus oligarthra* (Diesing, 1863) (Cestoda: Taeniidae) are the only two species known of Neotropical tapeworms, which cause Echinococcosis Polycystic (EP) and Echinococcosis Unicystic (EU), respectively, in humans and in wild rodents from Central and South America. This review applied a meta-analysis on published research about these diseases during the last decade (2010–2020) with the aim of finding out the new human cases reported on that decade on EP and EU. Several new human cases have been published in these 10 years, and important findings have been carried out on the phylogenetic taxonomy, on the genome of *E. oligarthra*, and on new molecular diagnostic techniques and imagenology applied upon this two neotropical echinococcosis, in particular in Argentina and Brazil. Finally, the life cycle of both *Echinococcus* species appears to be in a dynamic activity, apparently there is an expansion of both zoonotic diseases moving down to Southern zones of Argentina; therefore, a program of epidemiological surveillance on EP and EU is proposed to be carried out in those Patagonic regions.

Keywords: *Echinococcus vogeli*, *Echinococcus oligarthra*, echinococcosis, zoonosis

1. Introduction

Neotropical echinococcosis is a parasitic disease caused by two species of cestodes: *Echinococcus vogeli* (Rausch and Berstein, 1972) and *Echinococcus oligarthra* (Diesing, 1863), which are parasites in the small intestine of their specific definitive hosts: for *E. vogeli* the "bush dog" (*Speothos venaticus*, Lund, 1842), so far the only known natural host (some colloquial names for *S. venaticus* are: "pitoco dog" or "vinager fox" in Argentina; "cachorro do moto" in Brazil; "guache dog" in Venezuela and Colombia), whereas several species of wild cats (Felidae) are hosts for *E. oligarthra*. The life cycle of these two tapeworms follows the "predator-prey" seylvatic patron; thus, a wild rodent the paca (*Cuniculus paca*, Linnaeus, 1776) is the main known intermediate host for *E. vogeli* (the paca is named "lapa" in Venezuela; "guagua" in Colombia) even though it has also been collected from agouties (*Dasiprocta* spp., and from spiny rats (*Proechimis* spp.). On the other hand, metacestodes of *E. oligarthra*[1] have been found in tissues of several intermediate hosts such as the agouties [1] ("picures" in

1 *Echinococcus oligarthra*: new name given to the former species *Echinococcus oligarthrus*.

IntechOpen

Venezuela), spiny rats, pacas, opossums (*Didelphis marsupialis*), and in wild rabbits (*Sylvilagus floridanus*) [2] in tropical forests of Panama, Venezuela, Colombia, Chile, Brazil, and Argentina [3]. Proglotis and many eggs are shed from these tiny tapeworms into the gut lumen of their definitive hosts, passed out with the feces [4, 5], and next, eggs are accidentally ingested by the intermediate hosts, which become infected; in the case of *E. vogeli*, once in the intestine, the oncospheres stages are freed, invading organs such as the liver, lungs, small intestine, spleen, where develop they as protoscoleces, which asexually proliferate forming the hydatid polycystic cyst stage, polycystic for *E. vogeli*. The unicyst for *E. oligarthra* appears to be less erratic, and in three out of four cases diagnosed were found retrorbital. *Echinococcus oligarthra* was reported in its adult strobilar stage before 1860; nonetheless, more than 100 years (yr) have passed from the first report of the adult parasite to the recognition that this species infects humans causing the neotropical echinococcosis [6]. "Bush dogs" (*Speothos venaticus*) are less probably a direct source of infection for humans since it is a wild or seylvatic canid. On the contrary, hunting dogs (*Canis familiaris*), after being fed with raw viscera of pacas, are infected developing numerous Echinococcus *vogeli* cestodes in their small intestine, and thus in this way these dogs are the main responsible sources of infections for humans in rural zones. Therefore, *E. vogeli* and *E. oligarthra* metacestodes can have two transmission kinds of life cycles: (a) seylvatic and (b) rural or domestic to assure its survival as species [7].

A general taxonomic list for of these two *Echinococcus* tapeworms is as follows: Kingdom: Animalia; Phyum: Plathyelminthes; Class: Cestoda; Order: Cyclophylidea; Family: Taeniidae; Genus: *Echinococcus* (Rudolphi, 1801); and Neotropical species: *Echinococcus vogeli* and *E. chinococcus oligarthra* [6, 8]. On October 2019, the World Association of Echinococcosis (WAE) had its 28th World Cystic Echinococcosis Meeting at Lima, Peru, where it was updated the current nomenclature for the genus Echinococcus as follows: (a) it approved the names of Cystic Echinococcosis (for *E. granulosus*), Alveolar Echinococcosis (for *E. multilocularis*), and Neotropical Echinococcosis (for *E. vogeli*, and *E. oligarthra*), (b) the word "hydatid" from now on is used only for cysts caused by *E. granulosus sensu lato*, and (c) in the genus Echinococcus nine (09) species were officially recognized: *E. granulosus*, (*sensu lato* and *sensu stricto*), *E. multilocularis*, *E. canadiensis*, *E. equinus, E. felidis, E. ortleppi, E. shiquicus, E. vogeli*, and *E. oligarthra* [8].

The metacestodes of these two parasitic diseases are well documented and have been diagnosed in more than 200 people, mostly dwellers of tropical and subtropical areas from several Latin American Countries, (Nicaragua, Costa Rica, Panama, Colombia, Venezuela, Ecuador, Peru, Bolivia, Suriname, French Guiana, Paraguay, Brazil, Chile, Uruguay, and Argentina); these parasitoses are listed by the World Health Organization (WHO) among the 17 neglected tropical diseases and classified as zoonotic diseases [9]. The presence and impact of these neotropical parasitoses on humans in syelvatic and rural areas are directly related to different risk factors such as: (a) agricultural activities and deforestation, (b) continuing urbanization, (c) construction of new roads into syelvatic regions, (d) reduction of natural habits, (e) illegal hunting, plus capture and outlaw trade of wild animals, (f) infection in dogs due to their feeding with raw viscera, (g) possibility of scavenging dead animals, (h) lack of anthelmintic treatment, and (i) that these Neotropical Echinococcosis are not under surveillance and no compulsory official notification, because there is no obligation to report clinical cases in humans caused by these parasitic infections to health authorities in many countries of the region such as Colombia [10, 11] and also in other South American Countries [12–16]. The study of neotropical echinococcosis needs to follow and strengthen the holistic project of "One Health" following the WHO and the Pan American Health Organization (PAHO) plan of actions for hydatidosis for Latin American [9]. Therefore, a joint effort by veterinary and human medicine, environmental sciences, imagenology, and ecology is needed to improve our knowledge; in summary, it is a field that requires a multidisciplinary biomedical team to study its biology, diagnosis, treatment, surveillance, and control [3].

Few cases of human echinococcosis due to *E. oligarthra* infections have been diagnosed: the first case ever was a female patient from Venezuela who suffered a retroocular neotropical unicystic infection [17]; the second and third cases were diagnosed in Surinam showing one retroocular unicyst case, and another abdominal case [14, 18, 19]; the fourth case was a rural patient from Brazil who died of tetanus, and after necropsy an *E. oligarthra* unicystic stage was found at cardiac tissue [20]; and the fifth case was also in Brazil, and this patient had an hepatic neotropical unicyst infection [21]. On the contrary, in the period between 1979 and 2020. *E. vogeli* was responsible for causing more than 240 cases of human EP disease in several countries of Latin America [7, 22], and even few cases of EP have been diagnosed in the Netherlands from Suriname people who had moved to this European country [22]. The diagnosis of this neotropical echinococcosis originally has been carried out by the morphology of the cestodes shape, size, and length of the large and small rostellar hooks of these two Echinococcus cestodes [7]; however, the diagnosis has been widely improved in the last two decades: first, by the use of immunodiagnostic techniques such as ELISA, Western blot, or immunoeletrophoresis; second by molecular techniques (PCR) [22–26] and third by the use of imagenology equipment, i.e., ecography, including ultrasonography, Computerized Axial Tomography (CAT), Magnetic Resonance Imagenology (MRI), and conventional radiography; all are important for the diagnosis of CE; all these techniques are used not only for classification and identification of cysts, but also for monitoring the responses to treatments [7, 27–30]; consequently, the number of human cases diagnosed has increased, not only in new cases, but it has also been reported in countries where it had not been diagnosed, i.e., Peru [30, 31] and Argentina [32, 33]. In addition, in the Peruvian Amazon, a study was carried out in wild pacas looking for EP, and 11.7% of pacas were found to be infected with metacestodes of *E. vogeli*, thus representing these pacas' potential risks for humans living in that Peruvian region and for rural and urban dogs [3, 34].

2. Materials and methods

A meta-analysis was carried out as follows: articles search was performed by the author (RDM), since February 02, 2021, a systematic literature search was conducted on four databases to identify all publications reporting *Echinococcus vogeli, Echinococcus oligarthra*, Echinococcosis policystic, and Echinococcosis unicystic throughout the world in PubMed, Scopus, Research Gate, Google Scholar, and Medline, which were screened using those four (04) words without language restrictions.

Several inclusion criteria were required to meet articles to be selected: (a) should be scientific studies such as cross-sectional, longitudinal, case report or outbreak studies, published in indexed journals, reporting any natural infection of *E. vogeli* and/or *E. oligarthra*; (b) the study design, sample size, sample type, diagnostic methods, and number of *Echinococcus* infected animals; and (c) species of intermediate or definitive hosts animals for *E. vogeli* or/and *E. oligarthra* infections must be specified.

3. Results and discussion

The meta-analysis of scientific literature published between 2010 and 2020 showed that several new human cases of either neotropical EU and EP have been published during this decade, i.e.: (1) *Echinococcus vogeli* infection in a hunter from the rain forest of French Guiana was confirmed by imaging and mitochondrial Deoxyribonucleic Acid (DNA) sequence analysis [35]. (2) A case of infection by *E. oligarthra* in a Brazilian man was presented as a first case of Echinococcosis unicystic invasion of liver tissues [21]. (3) Two cases of liver EP were diagnosed by computerized tomography (CT) and ELISA in two female members of a Yanomani ethnic group located in the Amazonas State, Venezuela [36]. (4) Another human case of infection but by *E. vogeli* was reported from Argentina, the female patient was a Paraguayan immigrant who presented jaundice and abdominal pain in the right hypochondriac region. The diagnosis was achieved by abdominal CT, immunodiagnosis techniques (ELISA, immunoelectophoresis, Western blot), histopathologic studies, and molecular techniques (PCR) [37]. On the contrary, a review was recently published on the genus *Echinococcus* spp. [38], but new human clinical cases about neotropical EU and/or PE were not reported; the main information was about the life cycle and morphology of these two tapeworms [38].

The genus *Echinococcus* was recently studied through phylogenetic reconstructions of the relationship between several species using their mitochondrial DNA (mtDNA); moreover, molecular taxonomic analysis was also performed using short mtDNA sequences of genes for the cytochrome c oxidase subunit 1 (cox1) and for NAHD dehydrogenase subunit 1 (nad1) [39–41]. These studies concluded that the origin of the two species of Neotropical Echinococcus appears to be monophyletic; in other words, both share a common ancestor [42, 43]. This monophyletic result was more recently confirmed for *E. vogeli* after studies on its genetic diversity carried out in Western Brazilian Amazon [44, 45]. In addition, mitochondrial and nuclear sequence polymorphisms carried out with 38 isolates of *E. vogeli* from humans and wild animal hosts from Amazonian Regions revealed that *E. vogeli* is partially synanthropic, with a diverse population near or in association ecologically with humans [44, 45]. The use of molecular tools has shown differences in nucleic acid sequences that reflect phenotypic variation, and the phenotypic and genetic characteristics complement the previous observations published by the descriptive parasitologists years ago [20].

The genome of *E. oligarthra* was recently sequenced and assembled from hydatic unicysts obtained from tissues of an agouti (*Dasyprocta azarae*) [40], and it was estimated that its genome has a size of 86.2 megabases (Mb) and 8753 genes, which unexpectedly showed ~90% identity and 76.3% coverage with *Echinococcus multilocularis*, a tapeworm of Palearctic zones of the Northern hemisphere [46], and the phylogenetic work carried out on this *E. oligarthra* genome also showed that: (a) this neotropical genome is at a higher and farther distance from *E. granulosus*, and (b) *E. oligarthra* is one of the basal species of the genus *Echinococcus*. The genome size of *E. granulosus* was also recently estimated in 151.6 Mb, with 11,325 genes, and 9 pairs of chromosomes [47], therefore, the genome size of *E. oligarthra* is smaller, and almost half-size that of *E. granulosus*. The life cycle of *E. oligarthra* was also completed in the Upper Parana Atlantic Forest, Argentina, by microscopic, histological, and molecular techniques (PCR and nucleotide sequence of *E. oligarthra* DNA), and concluded that the agouti (*D. azarae*) is the main intermediate host (prey), and the felines Ocelot (*Leopardus pardalis*) and the puma (*Felis concolor*) are the definitive hosts of *E. oligarthra* [1, 32, 48].

It is considered that the number of human cases of neotropical unicystic and EP could be just "the tip of the iceberg" in relation to its real prevalence in Central and South America due to factors such as: (a) most infections occur to farmers, hunters, and rural people who lack medical assistance in those regions; (b) the development of these EP and EU cysts in human tissues or organs is slow and takes time, and during some years, patients are not aware of being parasitized by those polycysts; and (c) under those conditions patients are prone to suffer other infectious or organic diseases, which often might put an end to their lives. Therefore, the total number of human cases only for EP (232 for the year 2008) is perhaps only a small fraction of the real prevalence in South America countries, where there is lack of cumulative reports, of advanced diagnostic methods, and on-time treatment for EP [44]. In other clinical cases, parasitized farmers are able to obtain medical diagnosis and surgical treatment but with fatal results due to the advanced damage to organs such as the liver [21]. Previous publications showed that 172 human cases of Neotropical EU and EP were well documented from 12 countries in 2007 [7], whereas for the year 2008, a total of 232 similar cases were accounted, and from this last amount, 160 cases alone were diagnosed in Brazil (occurring in the States of Pará and Amapa, located in the Western Amazonian Region [44]. The difference between the 2007 and the 2008 data was 60 new cases, which means a 25.8% increment of new cases/year of Neotropical EU and EP per yr., if this percentage is taken as a reference point, then after 10 years (2010–2020), it may be estimated that at least more than 100 new cases of these parasitic diseases may have occurred in humans in seylvatic or rural regions, which were neither registered nor diagnosed.

The WHO included the EU and the EP among the 17 neglected tropical diseases and classified them as zoonotic diseases because these *Echinococcus* parasites infected humans in rural zones and seylvatic regions of Central and South America, where an early diagnosis and treatment for infected people are a difficult process. In this review it was stated that an exact cumulative annual number of human cases in the American Continent is lacking, due to the rural and remote origin of the patients, adults or teenagers, who get the fecal-oral infection from parasitized rural dogs or due to drinking water contaminated with feline feces. On the bases of the difference between the number of clinical cases of EP, published in 2007 and 2008 [7], it can be hypothesized that each year, between 2010 and 2020, may have occurred at least 10 new cases of human EP and of EU; unfortunately, none of those cases would have been registered in any hospital or medical services. Consequently, after a decade it may be estimated that no less than 100 humans were infected and suffered mainly EP. Nonetheless, a review of scientific literature for that decade shows that fewer than 100 human cases of these Neotropical echinococcoses have been published in journals, studied, diagnosed, and received medical services [20, 49].

4. Conclusions

It is important to underscore that *E. oligarthra* unexpectedly showed ~90% identity and 76.3% coverage with *Echinococcus multilocularis*, a tapeworm located in Palearctic zones of the Northern hemisphere, and this conclusion of genetic identity similarity can lead to hypothesize that *E. oligarthra* could have arrived to the American Continent through the Bering icy bridge. Next, it moved down this continent in the guts of some feline predators, then it crossed the Panama land isthmus millions of years ago arriving to Norther seylvatic lands of South America (now countries such as Colombia, Ecuador, and Venezuela), and nowadays, this *E. oligarthra* tapeworm appears to be still traveling down territories of the South Cone, perhaps heading toward Patagonia areas. The origin of the Neotropical echinococcosis showed that both tapeworms were brought to South America from North America. In the last year and for the first time, *E. oligarthra* was found, diagnosed, and its life cycle was completed in the Province of Misiones, north subtropical forest of Argentina. It may be hypothesized that both Neotropical *Echinococcus* still has a dynamic life cycle, which may be moving down toward some southern provinces of Argentina). Finally, a proposal would be to keep an epidemiological surveillance program in Southern provinces of Argentina as a public health action to figure out the presence or absence of these Neotropical echinococcoses in those Patagonic Regions.

Acknowledgements

Thanks to Consejo de Desarrollo Científico, Humanístico y Tecnológico (CDCHT) of Universidad Centroccidental Lisandro Alvarado (UCLA), Barquisimeto, Lara, Venezuela, for logistic and financial support upon this research.

Author details

Roy D. Meléndez
Universidad Centroccidental Lisandro Alvarado (UCLA), Decanato de Ciencias Veterinarias (DCV), Unidad de Investigación en Parasitología Veterinaria (UNIPARVET), Barquisimeto, Lara, Venezuela

*Address all correspondence to: empleomatic@gmail.com

References

[1] Zimmerman DM, Douglass M, Reavill DR, Greiner EC. *Echinococcus oligarthrus* cystic hydatidosis in Brazilian agouti (*Dasyprocta leporina*). Journal of Zoo and Wildlife Medicine. 2009;**40**:551-558

[2] Meléndez RD, Yépez MS, Coronado A. *Echinococcus oligarthrus* cysts of rabbits in Venezuela. The Journal of Parasitology. 1984;**70**:1004-1005

[3] Alessandro A. Polycystic echinococcosis in tropical America: *Echinococcus vogeli* and *E. oligarthrus*. Acta Tropica. 1997;**67**(1-2):43-65. DOI: 10.1016/s0001-706x(97)00048-x

[4] Batista Das Neves L, Ferlini-Teixeira PE, Silva S, de Bittencourt OF, García DD, de Barboza AF, et al. First molecular identification of *Echinococcus vogeli* and *Echinococcus granulosus* (*sensu stricto*) G1 revealed in feces of domestic dogs (*Canis familiaris*) from Acre, Brazil. Parasites and Vectors. 2017;**10**:28-34. DOI: 10.1186/s13071-016-1952-0

[5] Mehlhorn H. Echinococcus species: Tiny tapeworms. In: Strube CE, Mellhorn H, editors. Dog Parasites Endangering Human Health: Parasitology Research Monographs. Cham: Springer; 2021. p. 294

[6] Thompson RC. The taxonomy, phylogeny and transmission of Echinococcus. Experimental Parasitology. 2008;**119**:439-446. DOI: 10.1016/j.exppara.2008.04.016

[7] D'Alessandro A, Rausch RL. New aspects of neotropical policystic (*Echinococcus vogeli*) and unicystic (*Echinococcus oligarthrus*) Echinococcosis. Clinical Microbiology Review. 2008;**2**:380-401

[8] Vuitton DA, McManus DP, Rogan MT, Romig T, Gottstein B, Naidich A, et al. The World Association of Echinococcosis. International consensus on terminology to be used in the field of echinococcoses. Parasite. 2020;**27**:1-41. DOI: 10.1051/parasite/2020024

[9] WHO. Control of Neglected Tropical Diseases. Washington, USA: WHO; 2021

[10] Mondragon-Cardona AJ, Durán-Gutiérrez LF, Yucuma Gutiérrez S, Bolaños F, Vizcaychipi K, Alzate-Carvajal V, et al. Neotropical echinococcosis caused by *Echinococcus vogeli* in rural Huila, Colombia: Report of two last cases in the last 35 years. International Journal of Infectious Diseases. 2018;**73**(Suppl):306-307. DOI: 10.1016/i. ijid.2018.04.4112

[11] Rodríguez-Morales AJ, Calvo-Betancourt LS, Alarcón Olave C, Bolívar-Mejía A. Echinococcosis in Colombia. A neglected zoonosis? In: Current Topics in Echinococcosis. London: Intech; 2015. pp. 1-30

[12] Carmona D, Cardona GA. Echinococcosis in wild carnivorous species: Epidemiology, genotypic diversity, and implications for veterinary public health. Veterinary Parasitology. 2014;**202**(3-4):69-94. DOI: 10.1016/j.vetpar.2014.03.009

[13] Kumar K, Praveen PK, Ganguly S. Hydatidosis, a parasitic zoonotic disease: An overview. Review paper. International Journal of Science and Environmental Technology. 2016;**5**(5):3610-3614

[14] Oosturg BEJ, Eersel M, Vrede MA, Gottstein B, Rausch RL, D'Alessandro A. Preliminary field observations on

neotropical echinococcosis in Suriname. Revista de Patologia Tropical. 2004;**33**(1):125-134. DOI: 10.5216/rpt.v33i1.3252

[15] Otero-Abad B, Torgerson PR. A systematic review of the epidemiology of echinococcosis in domestic and wild animals. PLoS Neglected Tropical Diseases. 2013;**7**:2249

[16] Vizcaychipi KA, Rinas A, Irazu L, Miyagi A, Argüelles CF, Dematteo KE. Neotropical zoonotic parasites in bush dogs (*Speothos venaticus*) from upper Parana Atlantic forests in Misiones, Argentina. Vector-Born Zoonotic Diseases. 2016;**16**(10):664-672. DOI: 10.1089/vbz.2015.1929

[17] Lopera RD, Meléndez RD, Fernández I, Sirit J, Perera M. Orbital hydatid cyst of *Echinococcus oligarthrus* in a human in Venezuela. The Journal of Parasitology. 1989;**75**(3):467-470. DOI: 10.2307/328260

[18] Basset D, Girou C, Nizios IP, D'Hermies FD, Hoang C, Gordon R, et al. Neotropical echinococcosis in Suriname: *Echinococcus oligarthrus* in the orbit and *Echinococcus vogeli* in the abdomen. The American Journal of Tropical Medicine and Hygiene. 1989;**59**:787-790

[19] Debourgogne A, Blanchet D, Fior A, Umhang G, Somón S, Aznar C. Neotropical echinococcosis caused by Echinococcus vogeli in a 6-year-old child: The second case report in humans in French Guiana. Paediatric International Child Health. 2017;**37**:63-65. DOI: 10.1179/2046905515Y.0000000054

[20] Soares MC, Moreira-Silva CA, Nunes HM, Abraçado do Moral I, Pereira-Mória LJM, Silva-Conde SRS, et al. Equinococose policistica na Amazônia Oriental brasileira: acualizaçao da casuística. Revista da Sociedade Brasileira de Medicina Tropical. 2004;**37**(Suppl. 1):75-83

[21] Soares MC, Rodrigues AI, Moreira-Silva CA, Figuereido Brito EM, Gomes-Gouvéa MS, Dos Santos-Correia IR, et al. Anatomo-clinical and molecular description of liver neotropical echinococcosis caused by *Echinococcus oligarthrus* in human host. Acta Tropica. 2013;**125**(1):110-114

[22] Stijnis K, Dijkmans AC, Bart A, Brosens LA, Muntau B, Schoen C, et al. *Echinococcus vogeli* in immigrant from Suriname to the Netherlands. Emerging Infectious Diseases. 2015;**21**(3):528-530. DOI: 10.3201/eid2103.141205

[23] De la Rue M, Yamano K, Almeida CE, Lesbich MP, Fernandes C, Goto A, et al. Serological reactivity of patients with Echinococcus infections (*E. granulosus, E. vogeli, and E. multilocularis*) against three antigen B subunits. Parasitol. Résumé. 2010;**106**(3):741-745. DOI: 10.1007/s00436-009-1707-3

[24] Erdoğan E, Özkan B, Mutlu F, Karaca S, Sahin ML. Molecular characterization of *Echinococcus granulosus* isolates obtained from different hosts. Mikrobiyoloji Bülteni. 2017;**51**(1):79-86. DOI: 10.5578/mb.45452

[25] Siles-Lucas M, Gottenstein BB. Molecular tools for the diagnosis of cystic and alveolar echinococcosis. Tropical Medicine & International Health. 2001;**6**:463

[26] Siles-Lucas M, Casulli A, Conraths FJ, Meuller N. Laboratory diagnosis of Echinococcus spp. in human patients and infected animals. In: Thompson A, editor. Echinococcus Echinococcosis. Vol. 95. London, UK: Elsevier; 2017. pp. 159-257. DOI: 10.1016/bs.apar.2016.09.003

[27] Kern P, Menezes da Silva A, Akhan O, Müllhaupt B, Vizcaychipi KA, Budke C,

et al. The Echinococcoses: Diagnosis, clinical management and burden of disease. In: Deplazes P, Lymbery AJ, editors. Advanced: Parasitology. London, UK: Elsevier; 2017. pp. 259-369

[28] Meneghelli UG, Barbó ML, Magro JE, Bellucci AD, Llorach-Velludo MA. Polycystic hydatid disease (*Echinococcus vogeli*): Clinical and radiological manifestations and treatment with albendazole of a patient from the Brazilian Amazon region. Arquivos de Gastroenterologia. 1986;**23**:177

[29] Siqueiramn CM, Rodrígues-Silva R, Soares MC, Póvoa MM. Polycystic echinococcosis in the state of Acre, Brazil: Contribution to patient diagnosis, treatment and prognosis. Memórias do Instituto Oswaldo Cruz. 2013;**108**:533

[30] Somocurcio JR, Sánchez EL, Náquira C, Schidler J, Rojas F, Chacón P, et al. First report of a human case of polycystic echinococcosis due to *Echinococcus vogeli* from Neotropical area of Peru. South America. Revista do Instituto Medicina Tropical de São Paulo. 2004;**46**(1):41-42

[31] Zegarra A, Cáceres J, Piscoya A. 2010. Polycistic echinococcosis. Clinical Gastroenterology and Hepatology 8(10): E106. Doi: 10.1016/j.cgh.2010.02.018

[32] Arrabal JP, Avilab HG, Rivero MR, Camiciab F, Salas MM, Costa SA, et al. *Echinococcus oligarthrus* in the subtropical region of Argentina: First integration of morphological and molecular analyses determines two distinct populations. Veterinary Parasitology. 2017;**240**:60-67. DOI: 10.1016/j.vetpar.2017.03.019

[33] Vizcaychipi KA, Helou M, Dematteo K, Macchiarioli N, Cucher M, Rosenzvit M, et al. Primera identificación de *Echinococcus vogeli* en una paca en provincia de Misiones, Argentina. Revista Argentina de Microbiologia. 2013;**45**(3):169-173

[34] Mayor P, Baquedano LE, Sánchez E, Aramburu J, Gómez Puerta LA, Mamani VJ, et al. Polycystic echinococcosis in Pacas, Amazon Region, Perú. Emerging Infectious Diseases. 2015;**21**(3):456-459. DOI: 10.3201/eid2103.141197

[35] Knapp J, Chirica M, Simmonet C, Grenouillet F, Bart JM, Sako Y, et al. *Echinococcus vogeli* infection in a hunter, French Guiana. Emerging Infectious Diseases. 2009;**15**(12):2029-2031

[36] Noya-Alarcón O, Colmenáres C, Lander O, Montero M, Caltele H, Petit M, et al. Hidatidosis poliquística autóctona en dos pacientes Yanomami en el Alto Orinoco, Amazonas, Venezuela. Boletin de Malariologia Salud Ambiental. 2011;**51**(2):159-166

[37] Grenouillet F, Brider B, Álvarez-Rodríguez J, Amante M, Pestardo L, Cazorla A, et al. Molecular diagnosis of polycytic Echinococcosis due to *Echinococcus vogeli* in a Paraguayan immigrant in Argentina. Journal of Clinical Microbiology. 2013;**51**(9):3151-3153

[38] Brožova A, Jankovská I, Bejček V, Nechybová S, Peřinková P, Horáková S, et al. Echinococcus spp.: Tapeworms that pose a danger to both animals and humans: A review. Scientia Agriculturae Bohemica. 2017;**48**(4):193-201. DOI: 10.1515/sab-2017-0026

[39] Limbery AJ. Thylogenetic pattern, evolutionary process, and species delimitation in the genus Echinococcus. Advances in Parasitology. 2017;**95**:111-145

[40] Maldonado LL, Arrabal JP, Rosenzvit MC, Oliveira GCD,

KamenetzkyL. Revisitingthephylogenetic history of helminths through genomics, the case of the new *Echinococcus oligarthrus* genome. Frontiers in Genetics. 2019;**10**:708. DOI: 10.3389/fgene.2019.00708

[41] MacManus DP. Current status of the genetics and molecular taxonomy of Echinococcus species. Parasitology. 2013;**140**(13):1617-1623. DOI: 10.1017/S0031182013000802

[42] Nakao M, McManus DP, Schantz PM, Craig PS, Ito AA. Molecular phylogeny of the genus Echinococcus inferred from complete mitochondrial genomes. Parasitology. 2006;**134**:713

[43] Nakao M, Lavikainen A, Yanagida T, Ito A. Phylogenetic systematics of the genus Echinococcus (Cestoda: Taeniidae). Invited review. International Journal of Parasitology. 2013;**43**(12-13):1017-1029. DOI: 10.1016/j.ijpara.2013.06.002

[44] Daiper-García D, Galvao-Avan M, das Batista Neves L, Barbosa D, Almeida F, Ghiotti-Siqueira N, et al. Genetic diversity of *Echinococcus vogeli* in the Western Brazilian Amazon. Memorias do Instituto Oswaldo Cruz, Rio de Janeiro. 2019;**114**:1-4

[45] Santos GB, Soares M, Do CP, Brito M, André L, Rodrígues AL, et al. Mitochondrial and nuclear sequence polymorphisms reveal geographic structuring in Amazonian populations of *Echinococcus vogeli* (Cestoda: Taeniidae). International Journal for Parasitology. 2012;**42**:1115-1118

[46] Knapp J, Gottestein B, Saarma U, Millon L. Taxonomy, phylogeny and molecular epidemiology of *Echinococcus multilocularis*: From fundamental knowledge to health ecology. Veterinary Parasitology. 2015;**213**:85-91

[47] Zheng H, Zhang W, Zhang L, Zhang Z, Li J, Lu G, et al. The genome of the hydatid tapeworm *Echinococcus granulosus*. Nature Genetics. 2013;**45**(10):1168-1175. DOI: 10.1038/ng.2757

[48] Benatti D, de Santis M, Werther K, Tebaldi JH, Hoppe EGL. Helminth fauna of road-killed cougars (*Puma concolor*) from the Northeastern region of São Paulo State, Brazil. Brazilian Journal of Parasitology. 2021;**30**(1):570-574. DOI: 10.1590/S1984-29612021008

[49] Coyle CM. Polycystic Echinococcosis (Polycystic Neotropical Echinococcus). In: Ryan E, Hill D, Solomon T, Aronson N, Endy T, editors. Hunter's Tropical Medicine and Emerging Infectious Diseases. 10th ed. London, UK: Elsevier; 2019. 1264 pp. DOI: 10.1016/B978-0-323-55512-8.00134-4